Succeeding in the 2009 UK Clinical Aptitude Test (UKCAT)

Second edition

Matt Green
Jemini Jethwa

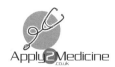

First published 2008
by Apply2 Ltd
Chelsea House
Chelsea Street
New Basford,
Nottingham, NG7 7HN
0800 6121135
www.Apply2Medicine.co.uk

Reprinted 2008

Second edition 2009

A catalogue record for this title is available from the British Library

ISBN 978-0-9556746-7-9

Typeset by Regent Typesetting, London
Printed by Bell and Bain, Glasgow

1 2 3 4 5 6 7 8 9 10

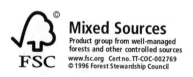

Mixed Sources
Product group from well-managed
forests and other controlled sources
www.fsc.org Cert no. TT-COC-002769
© 1996 Forest Stewardship Council

FSC

Testimonials from Previous Prospective Medical Students

'I found the guide really helpful and actually being able to practice the questions with the mock test really helped improved my confidence'

LS, Fife

'Thanks for all your help – the guide was excellent and would recommend it to anyone'

ND, Norwich

'I was really panicking about my UKCAT but your guide helped me prepare so that when I did the exam I was relaxed and knew what to expect – thankyou!'

PM, London

'Brilliant – No – Excellent guide. Would highly recommend it to anyone who wants to do well in their UKCAT'

CP, Nottingham

'Sat the UKCAT last week and I have to say that if I had not worked through your guide I would not have done nearly as well – will let you know my result when I get it'

MT, Cornwall

Acknowledgements

We would like to thank all those who provided such valuable feedback in relation to our UKCAT revision exercises.

Contents

About the Authors

Matt Green, BSc (Hons), MPhil

Matt Green, a former clinical scientist and founder of Apply2Medicine, has spent the last three years directly helping over 1,000 individuals prepare for and pass their UKCAT. It is with this extensive experience in mind that Matt has written this book to help prospective medical and dental students successfully pass the UKCAT as part of their application to university. Together with this title Matt has written books on Becoming a Doctor, Succeeding in the BMAT, Preparing your Medical School Application and Succeeding in the Medical School interview.

Jemini Jethwa, BSc (Hons), MSc

After completing a BSc in Human Psychology, Jemini went on to complete an MSc in Occupational Psychology at the University of Nottingham. Following extensive experience of compiling psychometric and aptitude tests over the course of her Masters degree, Jemini has been helping prospective medical and dentistry school students revise for the UKCAT since April 2007.

Preface

The aim of this book is to help you to prepare yourself fully for your approaching UKCAT. With the introduction of this test for the majority of UK Medical and Dental Schools, applicants need to ensure that they are more prepared than ever to succeed in their application.

This book addresses each of the five sections of the UKCAT, providing the reasoning behind each section of the test, together with example questions.

This guide culminates in an entire mock UKCAT test that you should complete under timed conditions. To gain the full benefit of this guide we recommend that you visit our website to download a free answer sheet to use when working through the example and mock test questions in this guide (www.apply2medicine.co.uk/ukcat). If you feel that you still require further practise after working through the examples and mock test contained within this guide, you can visit the Apply2Medicine website to subscribe to further online tests.

From all at Apply2Medicine we would like to wish you the best of luck with your application to Medical or Dental School.

Chapter 1

Introduction to the UKCAT

What is the UKCAT?

The UK Clinical Aptitude Test (UKCAT) is an aptitude test used as part of the selection process by a group of UK university Medical and Dental schools. The test has been devised in order to help universities further distinguish from the many applicants who apply for Medical or Dental programmes.

Candidates who apply to study Medicine or Dentistry will not only have to have excelled academically, they will also need to possess the relevant mental abilities, attitudes, views, perceptions and professional behaviours which are required of effective Doctors or Dentists.

The UKCAT provides universities with better information to enable them to select candidates of the highest calibre to progress successfully within the fields of Medicine or Dentistry. The UKCAT enables the elimination of unsuitable candidates at an early stage in the selection process, by testing for a number of skills and competencies, for example a candidate's ability to make decisions based on limited information.

The UKCAT, which is computer rather than paper-based, is coordinated by the UKCAT consortium in partnership with Pearson VUE, a global leader in computer based testing. The test is an 'on-screen test' and is delivered using a computer. The computer will time the test accordingly. Using this method of 'on-screen tests' is most convenient, as it allows the fast transfer of information to universities around the world. For security reasons you are unable to use your own personal computer and will need to use a computer at a designated test centre.

The test is delivered in locations across the globe through various Pearson high street centres. All applicants are encouraged to read carefully through the UKCAT website for specific guidance regarding registering for and sitting the test: www.ukcat.ac.uk

Content of the UKCAT

The UKCAT is a test of aptitude and is designed to measure general ability levels. The UKCAT does not test 'strict' academic or scientific knowledge. It assesses a certain range of mental abilities and behavioural attributes identified as being useful for healthcare professionals. Therefore it is easier to consider the UKCAT as a general ability IQ test or mental ability test.

The UKCAT is divided into five subtests:

1 **Verbal Reasoning** – assesses a candidate's ability to think logically about written information and to induce and deduce relevant conclusions

2 **Quantitative Reasoning** – assesses a candidate's ability to unravel numerical tasks

3 **Abstract Reasoning** – assesses a candidate's ability to deduce relationships using divergent and convergent thinking

4 **Decision Analysis** – assesses a candidate's ability to process an array of information to infer relationships, to formulate informed judgements and to decide on a correct response, in situations of intricacy and uncertainty

5 **Non-Cognitive Analysis** – identifies the traits and characteristics of robustness, integrity, honesty and empathy

Each of the above subtests are timed separately and comprise multiple choice questions and answers. You will be provided with a calculator by the test centre.

The total time allowed for the test is 120 minutes (which equates to 22 minutes each for the Verbal and Quantitative subtests, 16 minutes for the Abstract Reasoning subtest, 30 minutes for the Decision Analysis subtest, and a maximum of 30 minutes for the Non-Cognitive subtest). The times include a minute of preparation/administration time for each subtest. The preparation time is short because you are supposed to have familiarised yourself with the tests, and the format, before taking them.

The scaled scores for the first four subtests can range from 300 to 900. The majority of candidates score between 500 and 700, with the average score being 600. The results of the Non-Cognitive subtest will be reported in the form of a short description, and are used to indicate personal attributes and various characteristics related to successful careers within Medicine and Dentistry. It is important to note that the UKCAT does not have a pass rate. Your UKCAT results are used together with other factors, such as your Personal Statement and predicted grades, as an overall indicator of your suitability for a career in Medicine or Dentistry. Each University sets it own parameters as to how and to what degree the UKCAT results are used as part of the selection process. For example, some Universities rank candidates based on the subtest with the lowest score whereas others base their decision on the average score of the candidate.

Eligibility for the UKCAT

The UKCAT was formally adopted in 2006 and is now used by 26 Medical and Dental Schools in the UK (listed below). The requirement for applicants to complete the UKCAT applies to all UK, EU and the majority of international applicants. Test centres exist worldwide, including in most EU countries. Registration for the test is made online at www.ukcat.ac.uk.

Registering for the UKCAT

Registration for the 2009 UKCAT starts at the beginning of May 2009 via an online process. We would strongly recommend that you strive to sit the UKCAT at a time that does not impact on your studies if applicable, ideally during the summer. There is also an incentive of the test fee being reduced if you complete the test before the end of August 2009. If you do not take the UKCAT test before the deadline, your application will be automatically rejected, and you will have to reapply the following year.

Candidates who are intending to apply in 2009 for entry to the following Universities in 2010 or for deferred entry in 2011 are required to complete the UKCAT before the middle of October 2009 (exact date can be confirmed on the UKCAT website). The results from your test are only valid in the year the test is taken. If your application to Medicine or Dentistry is not successful and you re-apply the following year, you will have to re-sit the UKCAT.

If you have any special circumstances, such as a disability or illness, you may be provided with extra time to complete the test. However, you will need to give details of such circumstances at the time of registration, and provide evidence to substantiate this. There are two versions of the UKCAT, the Standard and the Special Educational Needs (SEN) version, which is the same test with extra time allowed for completion.

List of participating universities for the UKCAT

University of Aberdeen
Brighton and Sussex Medical School
Barts and The London School of Medicine and Dentistry
Cardiff University

University of Dundee
University of Durham
University of East Anglia
University of Edinburgh
University of Glasgow
Hull York Medical School
Keele University
King's College London
Imperial College London Graduate Entry
University of Leeds
University of Leicester
University of Manchester
University of Newcastle
University of Nottingham
University of Oxford Graduate Entry
Peninsula College of Medicine and Dentistry
Queen's University Belfast
University of Sheffield
University of Southampton
University of St Andrews
St George's, University of London
Warwick University Graduate Entry

How do I prepare?

Although it is stated that you cannot prepare for the UKCAT, this is simply not the case. Through completing practice tests you will have a clearer idea of what to expect and feel more confident. We would encourage you to read carefully through the UKCAT website so that you have a clear understanding of the test process and the interface that is used in the test centre.

To ensure that you are fully prepared for your UKCAT, work through this book and practise what you have learnt by completing the mock test (see Chapter 8) under timed conditions. The first part of this guide explains each sub-test of the UKCAT, why it used and provides practice questions for you to work through to ensure that you put into practice what you have learnt.

The second part of this guide comprises a full mock test that you can work through under timed conditions.

We would recommend that you visit our website to download our free answer sheet, which will make it easier to refer your answers back to the guide. There are also further mock tests available on our website.

Chapter 2

Succeeding in the UKCAT

Practice makes perfect

As with any test it is essential to practise example questions to ensure you are familiar with the structure and type of content you will be tested on. The UKCAT is no exception despite what people may tell you!

The following chapters will enable you to practise each of the different subtests which together form the UKCAT. Each chapter contains questions equivalent to half of what you would be faced with in the test, designed to help you to put into practice what you learn. This will enable you to familiarise yourself with the format and style of the UKCAT and hopefully help you to realise that most of the questions in the test will be of general ability.

However, this is not to say that the UKCAT test is of an easy nature, otherwise it would not be a useful tool in the selection process. Although the UKCAT may measure general ability you will find that you only have a limited amount of time for each subtest.

Each of the subtests is individually timed, therefore it is not possible for you to make up for lost time in the other remaining subtests. It is vital that you complete each section fully as you progress through the test and do not leave any questions unanswered. By doing so, if you find that you do not have time to go back and check your answers, you will at least stand a chance of scoring a mark.

It may therefore be more valuable to time yourself when you undertake the mock test at the end of this book. This will enable you to enhance your time management skills, increase your confidence and also alleviate any anxiety you may have. The aim of this book is to ensure that, on the day of your test, you are faced with something you are already familiar with.

This book culminates with a full mock test for you to complete under timed conditions. To help you make the most of this book, an answer sheet can be downloaded for free from www.apply2medicine.co.uk/UKCAT.

What are multiple choice tests?

The UKCAT is set out in a multiple choice format. Multiple choice tests are commonly used within the field of selection and assessment. The test questions are designed to test a candidate's awareness and understanding of a particular subject.

The subtests within the UKCAT are based on an answer format known as 'A-Type Questions', which is the most commonly used design in multiple choice tests. This specific design helps to make transparent the number of choices which need to be selected. These questions usually consist of a 'Stem and lead-in question' which are followed by a 'series' of 'choices'. To illustrate this, below is an example of a Quantitative Reasoning question:

Stem

This is generally an introductory statement, question or passage of relevant information which elicits the correct answer. The stem on the whole provides all the information for the question or questions which will follow, e.g.

   'There are 100 students who go on a school trip to a science park.'

Lead-in Question

This is the question which identifies the exact answer, e.g.

   'If 35% of the students were female, how many female students were there?'

Choices

In a multiple choice test, the choices will generally consist of one correct answer. However, depending on the type of question, you may be required to select two or even three correct answers. Wherever there are correct answers there are also incorrect answers, which are also known as the 'distracters'. For the above example, typical choices could be as follows:

A. 25

B. 67

C. 35 – Correct answer (35% of 100 students = 35 female students)

D. 65

General tips for answering multiple choice tests

- Read, and **re-read the question** to ensure you fully understand what is being asked, not what you want to be asked.

- Try to answer the question before looking at the choices available to you.

- **Eliminate any incorrect answers** you know are wrong.

- **Do not spend too much time on one question** – remember you only have a set amount of time per section so, as a rule of thumb, you should spend x amount per question (x = time of section ÷ number of questions).

- **Do not keep changing your mind** – research has shown that the first answer that appeals to you is often the correct one.

- If you cannot decide between two answers, look carefully and decide whether for one of the options you are making an unnecessary assumption – **trust your gut instinct.**

- Always select an answer for a given question even if you do not know the answer – **never leave any answers blank.**

- **Pace yourself** – you will need to work through the test at the right speed. Too fast and your accuracy may suffer, too slow and you may run out of time. Use this guide to practise your time keeping and approach to answering each question – you need to do what works for you, not what might work for someone else.

- In the actual test, you will be given the opportunity to mark your questions for review, so do try to remember and **go back and check** that you have answered all the questions to the best of your ability.

- To familiarise yourself with the way the online test will be conducted visit the **online testing demonstration** which is available on the UKCAT website.

- Remember you will only be awarded marks for correct answers, and marks will not be deducted for incorrect answers. Therefore try to **answer every single question**, even ones you are unsure of.

- When you take the test, listen carefully to the administrator's instructions.

- If you are unsure about anything, remember to ask the test administrator before the test begins. Once the clock begins ticking, interruptions will not be allowed.

- You may be presented with a question which you simply cannot answer due to difficulty or if the wording is too vague. If you have only 20 seconds per question, and you find yourself spending five minutes determining the answer for each question then your time management skills are poor and you are wasting valuable time.

Chapter 3

The Verbal Reasoning Subtest

The purpose of the UKCAT Verbal Reasoning subtest is to assess a candidate's ability to read and critically evaluate passages of written information which cover a variety of topics, including both scientific and non-scientific themes. The Verbal Reasoning subtest used in the UKCAT is a classic critical thinking and reasoning test. Critical reasoning and critical thinking are core skills which are required to achieve understanding of complex arguments, evaluate different perceptions and find solutions to problems.

Achieving high scores in the Verbal Reasoning subtest reflects a candidate's ability to interpret written information within the workplace based on the facts you are presented with, rather than letting your personal knowledge influence your decision, an essential skill required when working within a healthcare setting.

The following qualities are required to enable effective critical thinking and critical reasoning:

- The ability to differentiate between fact and opinion.

- The ability to examine and differentiate between assumptions, both those presented in the text and your own.

- The ability to be open minded but also flexible as you explore explanations, causes and solutions to various problems – without your own bias.

- Awareness of misleading arguments, which consist of vague and manipulative reasoning.

- The ability to remain focused on the overall picture while investigating specifics based on the information present.

- The ability to discover reputable sources.

The Verbal Reasoning subtest in the UKCAT consists of 11 stems or passages of written information. Each passage comprises four lead-in questions/statements, which in total equal 44 items to complete. For each answer you will have three options: 'True', 'False' or 'Can't tell'. You will be allocated 22 minutes to complete this section, which includes one minute administration time, which equates to 30 seconds per question.

For each of the stems, you will be faced with a passage which has been extracted from various sources. These passages do not contain any curriculum content. However, the purpose of each of the passages is to try and persuade the reader to adopt a specific view of an argument. **The key to approaching Verbal Reasoning questions is to base your decision purely on the information and facts provided in the passages**. You must avoid using any previous knowledge you may have regarding each subject to bias your answer. The aim of the Verbal Reasoning subtest is to read the passage, and evaluate the four corresponding statements, according to the following rules:

True – if you consider the statement to be true based on the information provided in the passage.

False – if you consider the statement to be false based on the information provided in the passage.

Can't tell – if you cannot state whether the statement is true or false without further information which is not provided.

Summary of Verbal Reasoning structure

Stem

The stem will consist of a series of passages, extracted from various different sources such as leaflets, magazines, newspaper articles, and various other sources of written information. The Verbal Reasoning subtest consists of 11 stems.

Lead-in question

Each of the stems will consist of four separate lead-in questions which are related to the stem in some way. Therefore there will be a total of 44 lead-in questions.

Choices

Your task will be to decide whether the lead-in question is 'True', 'False' or 'Can't tell' based purely on the evidence given in the passages or stems.

Time limit = 22 minutes. Therefore you will have 30 seconds per question.

When you are working through the UKCAT subtests it can be counter-productive to monitor exactly how long you spend on answering each question, especially when you need to read through and digest the information presented in the stem. Therefore a more useful time management approach is to divide each subtest into four quarters. So, in the case of the Verbal Reasoning subtest, after approximately six minutes you should be working on the fourth passage, after approximately 11 minutes you should be commencing the seventh passage and so on. If you find yourself falling behind at these points you know that you need to pick up the pace.

Example of a Verbal Reasoning question

> It has been a controversial debate that half of the jobs which Labour created in 1997 have been filled by foreign workers. The Department of Work and Pensions claims that over 52% of jobs have gone to foreign workers. One recent 'eye-opener' has been that the government has declared that more than 1.1 million overseas workers have come to Britain in the past 10 years, and not 8 million as previously disclosed.
>
> National statistics provided by the Home Office indicate that 1.5 million overseas workers have entered the UK over the last decade. However, in reply to this the Department of Work and Pensions has claimed that the extra 400,000 workers were British residents who were born overseas. With such statistics the findings seem to make a mockery of what the government had initially proposed – 'British jobs for every British worker'.

A   48% of jobs have gone to British workers.

   Answer: True, False or Can't tell

Verbal Reasoning hints and tips

- **Ensure the answer you give is determined solely by the information contained within the passage and not your assumptions.**

- Look out for misleading words such as '*all*', '*everything*' and '*completely*' – these are specific types of words which suggest that the whole of a particular object, person, area or group are wholly affected.

- Other misleading words include '*virtually*', '*almost*', '*particularly*', '*nearly*' and '*close to*' – these are words which refer to something *close to* happening rather than actually happening.

- It is important that you **read the passages very carefully**. One common mistake that candidates often make is to allow their previous knowledge on a subject to interfere with and bias the information and facts that are presented in the passages (often these are of a conflicting nature).

- Remember that each of the passages is **deliberately manipulated to influence the candidate** to a particular perspective or point of view.

- Often you may find that a passage states information which may subsequently alter or be contradicted further on in the passage. Ensure that you note any changes or contradictions and reflect these when selecting your answers.

- **Do not waste too much time thinking about a difficult question**. All questions are marked equally, therefore a difficult question will not be worth more than an easy question and vice versa. If you are having difficulty understanding a passage, flag it and move on to the next passage, ensuring that you come back to it later.

- Remember **time management is key throughout** the test and in the Verbal Reasoning subtest you should spend no longer than 30 seconds considering an answer.

- If you find a question particularly difficult you can flag it so that you can return to it before you move on to the next subtest – when flagging a question to return to we recommend that you still select an answer in case you do not have time to return to the question.

- **Attempt all questions** as you will not be penalised for getting questions wrong, but you will lose marks if you leave an answer blank.

- Learn to **manage your time efficiently**. Go through practice mock papers and time yourself as if you were in a real exam. By familiarising yourself with the types of questions you will be faced with you will be able to analyse where your weaknesses are and improve.

- Read through newspapers and various other sources of literature which use elaborate and detailed language. This will enhance your skills in reading and also enable you to consider in-depth critical arguments and perspectives.

Seven simple steps to Verbal Reasoning

Step 1

Browse through the passages (answering each question systematically) and try to gain a feel for what the passage is trying to portray. Remember not to let previous knowledge on a subject interfere with what is actually presented in the passage.

Step 2

Note down any changes or contradictions in terms of information or valid points.

Step 3

Read through each question and determine exactly what you are being asked.

Step 4

Read through the passage again if necessary and answer each of the questions. Remember to take into account previous notes.

Step 5

Eliminate answers which are obviously incorrect.

Step 6

Try to answer the questions as accurately as possible and do not leave any answers blank, even if you are not sure of the answer.

Step 7

If you are having trouble answering any of the questions, still select an answer and flag it so you can return to it later.

Verbal Reasoning practice examples

The following part of this chapter will enable you to work through various examples of Verbal Reasoning questions together with evaluating your answers against explanations. Remember, you can download a free answer sheet from www.apply2medicine.co.uk to make it easier for you when working through these examples.

Example1

> *From the beginning it was evident that the project was ambitious in size, intricacy and in its pioneering development of the Finance and Insurance initiatives. It was obvious that the project was going to be complex and most certainly difficult and this is what had contributed towards the failure of the project's development. However, if the estimation of the timescales and the level of difficulty had been more cautiously considered, the department may have been able to evaluate the virtues of the project more effectively.*
>
> *In July 2006, 'Phoenix 2' indicated that they required an extension to complete the project – this requirement was most foreseeable. If the department had questioned the required timescale, difficulty and complexity then the halt may have been avoided. It is questionable whether the department had considered inception, especially making an allowance for the implications of setback on the business case on their scheme.*

A   If the department had been more prudent when estimating the difficulty of the project, the project would not have failed.

B   Phoenix 2 withheld information regarding the timescale of the project, as they knew it was going to be a difficult task.

C   The department's profits were dependent upon the length of the project.

D   The department was unaware of the ambiguity and complexity of the project.

Example 2

> *Theoretically speaking, both industrial consumers and private households are now able to openly select their energy supplier following the entry into force of (European Union) EU directives in 2004 and 2007. However, many hindrances remain within a single European energy market which makes it a far cry from reality. To compensate for the shortcomings, the European Commission has proposed to inflate 'Energy Market Liberalisation'. The commission suggests that gas and electricity companies unbundle their ownership of power grids and pipelines to augment competition. Foreign companies would also have to unbundle their ownership, if they wanted to enter the market. This may seem like a warning to Russia's Gazprom, who supply 25% of the gas to Europe. Another issue with the proposal is that some EU countries have not yet completely released their electricity and gas markets to competition, thereby effectively blocking new business from entering the market and bringing the prices down.*

A   Financial incentives play no part in the development of 'Energy Market Liberalisation'.

B   Gas and electricity companies have to sell their products and services separately rather than in a combined form.

C   The 'Energy Market Liberalisation' will increase competition between various companies.

D   The objectives of the directives are to open up electricity and gas markets through competition, thereby increasing the overall efficiency of the energy sector.

Example 3

> *Ever since the gun was invented, it has transformed the way the world thinks, in several ways. Many of these changes have been brought about by mans' yearning for self-protection. For every key development of the gun, there has been an important consequence for the world. The gun has enabled the discovery of the world and the development of society.*
>
> *In recent years there has been a serious outcry about the use of weapons amongst worldwide gang cultures. These gangs generally comprise men and women, adults and adolescents. There have been numerous accounts of gang members using various weapons. Gang members who have weapons are often perceived as individuals with high status and authority.*

A   The gun was invented to protect mankind.

B   Gang members with guns are considered to be people with high status.

C   Guns have made society the way it is today.

D   Guns have made humankind think about self-protection.

Example 4

> The British Medical Association has been very concerned with regards to children's health and nutrition. Childhood obesity rates are continually increasing dramatically. This is extremely worrying as obesity can cause various life-threatening diseases such as heart disease, osteoarthritis and some cancers. The government has noticed this increase in obesity and has gradually begun to promote healthy eating. For example, food labelling has been introduced in order to help individuals realise the unnecessary fats, sugars and salt levels they are taking in on a regular basis. However, the problem with some schools is that they are finding it difficult to serve nutritious food on tight budgets.

A   School meals would improve if the schools had more money.

B   Obesity rates are higher now than in previous years.

C   Children who eat healthily will suffer less from heart disease, osteoarthritis and cancers.

D   Schools are finding it difficult to serve good food as they are on tight budgets.

Example 5

> Since the beginning of the early 1980s, the British Medical Association (BMA) has called for a total ban on amateur and professional boxing within the UK. The BMA have called for this ban based on medical evidence which suggests that boxing not only causes acute injury, but can also cause chronic brain damage which is sustained cumulatively. The BMA has stated that modern medical technology demonstrates, without hesitation, that chronic brain damage is caused by recurrent blows to the head, which all boxers will experience from being in the ring.

A   Amateur and professional boxers will experience blows to the head.

B   Acute injury is sustained gradually.

C   The effects of brain damage are gradually built up.

D   Modern technology can scan brain damage.

Justifications of Verbal Reasoning practice examples

Example 1

> *From the beginning it was evident that the project was ambitious in size, intricacy and in its pioneering development of the Finance and Insurance initiatives. It was obvious that the project was going to be complex and most certainly difficult and this is what had contributed towards the failure of the project's development. However, if the estimation of the timescales and the level of difficulty had been more cautiously considered, the department may have been able to evaluate the virtues of the project more effectively.*
>
> *In July 2006, 'Phoenix 2' indicated that they required an extension to complete the project – this requirement was most foreseeable. If the department had questioned the required timescale, difficulty and complexity then the halt may have been avoided. It is questionable whether the department had considered inception, especially making an allowance for the implications of setback on the business case on their scheme.*

A   *If the department had been more prudent when estimating the difficulty of the project, the project would not have failed.*

Answer: True

In the passage it is stated 'If the estimation of the timescales and the level of difficulty had been more cautiously considered, the department may have been able to evaluate the virtues of the project more effectively'. Following this statement, it is evident that if the department had been slightly more cautious (or prudent) and evaluated the merits of the project more effectively, the project may have been a success.

B   *Phoenix 2 withheld information regarding the timescale of the project, as they knew it was going to be a difficult task.*

Answer: Can't tell

There is no information in the passage which suggests that Phoenix 2 withheld information regarding the timescale of the project. The only information on the topic of timescale is that the department required an extension.

C   *The department's profits were dependent upon the length of the project.*

Answer: True

This statement is true as it is proposed in the passage that the 'business case', (which is a business plan that forecasts costs and profits for the project) was set back.

D   **The department was unaware of the ambiguity and complexity of the project.**

Answer: Can't tell

In the passage the author writes in the third person that it was inevitable that the project was going to be complex. However there is no information in the passage which states whether or not the department knew itself that the project was going to be ambiguous.

Example 2

> *Theoretically speaking, both industrial consumers and private households are now able to openly select their energy supplier following the entry into force of European Union (EU) directives in 2004 and 2007. However, many hindrances remain within a single European energy market which makes it a far cry from reality. To compensate for the shortcomings, the European Commission has proposed to inflate 'Energy Market Liberalisation'. The commission suggests that gas and electricity companies unbundle their ownership of power grids and pipelines to augment competition. Foreign companies would also have to unbundle their ownership, if they wanted to enter the market. This may seem like a warning to Russia's Gazprom, who supply 25% of the gas to Europe. Another issue with the proposal is that some EU countries have not yet completely released their electricity and gas markets to competition, thereby effectively blocking new business from entering the market and bringing the prices down.*

A   Financial incentives play no part in the development of 'Energy Market Liberalisation'.

Answer: Can't tell

There is no information in the passage which suggests that the Energy Market Liberalisation was introduced with an aim of financial incentives or profits. However it is stated within the passage that there are 'shortcomings', but we are not given information about whether these shortcomings are specifically related to financial aspects.

B   Gas and electricity companies have to sell their products and services separately rather than in a combined form.

Answer: True

In the passage it is stated 'The commission suggests that gas and electricity companies *unbundle* their ownership of power grids and pipelines to augment competition'. Unbundle simply means to sell or charge for products as single items rather than in a combined form. Therefore the statement is true.

C   *The 'Energy Market Liberalisation' will increase competition between various companies.*

Answer: Can't tell

The above statement indicates that there *will* be a definite increase in competition, however in the passage the Energy Market Liberalisation is in fact a proposal. It is not a legislation which has already been enforced, hence the effects of the legislation are still unknown.

D   *The objectives of the directives are to open up electricity and gas markets through competition, thereby increasing the overall efficiency of the energy sector.*

Answer: Can't tell

The main body of the passage simply gives information about the actual proposal itself and not the objectives and justifications for these upcoming proposals. Hence there is limited information to conclude the statement above.

Example 3

> *Ever since the gun was invented, it has transformed the way the world thinks, in several ways. Many of these changes have been brought about by mans' yearning for self-protection. For every key development of the gun, there has been an important consequence for the world. The gun has enabled the discovery of the world and the development of society.*
>
> *In recent years there has been a serious outcry about the use of weapons amongst worldwide gang cultures. These gangs generally comprise men and women, adults and adolescents. There have been numerous accounts of gang members using various weapons. Gang members who have weapons are often perceived as individuals with high status and authority.*

A   The gun was invented to protect mankind.

Answer: Can't tell

There is no information in the passage which justifies reasons why the gun was invented. We may personally know why the gun may be used; however it is important not to confuse our personal knowledge with what is actually stated in the passage.

B   Gang members with guns are considered to be people with high status.

Answer: True

In the passage it suggests that gang members who carry *weapons* are considered to be perceived as having high authority.

C   Guns have made society the way it is today.

Answer: False

The above statement is incorrect, as it is proposed in the passage that guns have *enabled the discovery of* the world and developed society rather than made society the way it is today.

D   Guns have made humankind think about self-protection.

Answer: False

In the passage it is suggested that the gun has changed the way the world thinks, but 'Many of these changes have been brought about by mans' yearning for self-protection'. Therefore the concept of 'self-protection' has been ever present.

Example 4

> *The British Medical Association has been very concerned with regards to children's health and nutrition. Childhood obesity rates are continually increasing dramatically. This is extremely worrying as obesity can cause various life-threatening diseases such as heart disease, osteoarthritis and some cancers. The government has noticed this increase in obesity and has gradually begun to promote healthy eating. For example, food labelling has been introduced in order to help individuals realise the unnecessary fats, sugars and salt levels they are taking in on a regular basis. However, the problem with some schools is that they are finding it difficult to serve nutritious food on tight budgets.*

A   *School meals would improve if the schools had more money.*

Answer: Can't tell

It is stated in the passage that some schools are having problems with funding for healthier meals; however there is no information which suggests that the school meals would actually improve if they had more money.

B   *Obesity rates are higher now than in previous years.*

Answer: True

In the passage it is stated that '*Childhood obesity rates are continually increasing dramatically*'. Therefore the obesity rates have been continuous over the years and hence are higher than in previous years.

C   *Children who eat healthily will suffer less from heart disease, osteo-arthritis and cancers.*

Answer: Can't tell

In the passage there is information about the effects of obesity, however there is no information which explains what the effects of healthy eating are.

D   *Schools are finding it difficult to serve good food as they are on tight budgets.*

Answer: False

The above statement is false as it generalises that 'all' schools are finding it difficult to serve good food due to tight budgets, when in fact there are 'some' schools that are finding it difficult to fund for healthy eating.

Example 5

> *Since the beginning of the early 1980s, the British Medical Association (BMA) has called for a total ban on amateur and professional boxing within the UK. The BMA have called for this ban based on medical evidence which suggests that boxing not only causes acute injury, but can also cause chronic brain damage which is sustained cumulatively. The BMA has stated that modern medical technology demonstrates, without hesitation, that chronic brain damage is caused by recurrent blows to the head, which all boxers will experience from being in the ring.*

A   *Amateur and professional boxers will experience blows to the head.*

Answer: True

It is implied in the passage that 'all' boxers will experience blows to the head, therefore it is correct to generalise that it will affect both amateur and professional boxers.

B   *Acute injury is sustained gradually.*

Answer: Can't tell

In the passage it is suggested that boxing does cause acute injury; however there is no information which suggests that these injuries are sustained gradually.

C   *The effects of brain damage are gradually built up.*

Answer: True

It is suggested within the passage that brain damaged is sustained 'cumulatively' – which simply means it is gradually built up.

D   *Modern technology can scan brain damage.*

Answer: Can't tell

It is stated within the passage that modern technology is able to show that chronic brain damage is caused by boxing. However there is no information which suggests that modern technology specifically 'scan' for brain damage.

Chapter 4

The Quantitative Reasoning Subtest

The Quantitative Reasoning subtest of the UKCAT will assess a candidate's ability to solve numerical problems, interpret data and also assess their basic maths skills relating to real life scenarios. The aim of this subtest is to objectively assess a candidate's ability to analyse, interpret, and manipulate complex numerical data.

Achieving high scores in the Quantitative Reasoning subtest reflects a candidate's ability to manipulate numerical information, which is an essential skill required by Doctors or Dentists in their everyday practice.

Before you attempt to answer any Quantitative Reasoning questions it is important that you refresh your basic knowledge of the following topics:

- Addition
- Subtraction
- Multiplication
- Division
- Percentages
- Ratio
- Mean, median and mode
- Fractions
- Decimal numbers

Also, you need to be able to interpret:

- Pie charts
- Line Graphs

- Bar graphs

- Tables

The Quantitative Reasoning subtest contains 10 stems comprising various tables, charts and graphs, with a total of 40 questions relating to them (four items per stem). You will have 22 minutes to complete this section which includes one minute for administration. You will therefore have 33 seconds to complete each question.

This chapter will illustrate various examples of the types of numerical questions you will face when you sit your UKCAT.

Summary of Quantitative Reasoning structure

Stem

The stem will consist of various tables, charts and graphs. There will be a total of 10 stems in the UKCAT.

Lead-in Question

For each of the stems, there will be four separate lead-in questions. In total there will be 40 lead-in questions which relate to the various charts, graphs and tables.

Choices

You will be given five different answer options which will be in the format of A, B, C, D and E. Only one choice is the correct answer, and the remaining choices are known as 'distracters'.

Time limit = 22 minutes. Therefore you will have 33 seconds per question.

When you are working through the UKCAT subtests it can be counter-productive to monitor exactly how long you spend on answering each question, especially when you need to read through and digest the information presented in the stem. Therefore a more useful time management approach is to divide each subtest into four quarters. So, in the case of the Quantitative Reasoning subtest, after approximately six minutes you should be working on the fifth stem, after approximately 11 minutes you should be commencing the tenth stem and so on. If you find yourself falling behind at these points you know that you need to pick up the pace.

Example of a Quantitative Reasoning question

Examine the table below

	Currency Rate of exchange = Pounds Sterling (£1)
American – Dollar	$1.59
Indian – Rupee	0.0856 R
French – Euro	1.45 €
Cuban – Peso	1.8 CUP
Bangladeshi – Taka	0.6 BGL

How much is $150 worth in Pounds Sterling (£)?

A £94.33

B £49.36

C £94.34

D £49.37

E £94.30

Quantitative Reasoning hints and tips

Refresh your memory by working through your GCSE and A level maths books to ensure you are familiar with the following:

- Addition and subtraction
- Multiplication and division
- Fractions and percentages
- Converting fractions, decimals and percentages
- Determining modes, means and medians
- Algebra
- Decimals
- Distance, time and speed triangles
- Calculating area and perimeters
- Analysing charts, bar charts, pie charts, frequency tables etc
- Square and cube numbers

- **Work through the questions systematically.** You may find that a question refers to your previous answer(s).

- **Work out all your calculations on the whiteboard provided.** If there are errors you may be able to determine from your rough workings at what point you made a mistake.

- Go through the practice mock papers and **identify your strengths and weaknesses** early so you can improve on your weaknesses. For example, you may be better at completing algebra equations rather than fractions. You can then address your weaknesses.

- When answering questions which involve humans, remember to calculate your final answer to the nearest whole number as people cannot be represented as a decimal or a fraction! This may be an important point to take note of when converting percentages to actual numbers.

- One major pitfall is to select an option which you think is nearest to the answer. Often you will find that the majority of the options are very close to each other and may differ in terms of decimal points or a single digit which is either added or removed. Therefore it is very important to evaluate the answer options very carefully.

- Always answer questions in the correct metric units. For example, a question may ask you to calculate something in centimetres but then give your final answer in metres. Therefore it is important to **read each item very carefully.**

- Some algebra questions may require you to calculate the value of 'x'. Often this will be x on its own or sometimes the answer may require you to find x^3 or x^2. Therefore it is always important to **look at how the questions require you to give your final answer.**

- Remember to **time yourself as you complete the mock tests**. This will improve your time management skills, ensuring you have adequate time to answer every question.

- Try not to spend too long on one question. All marks are awarded equally in this section. If you are unsure of the answer select the best possible answer, flag the question and return to it. By selecting an answer you at least stand a chance of scoring a mark, even if you run out of time and are unable to return to the flagged question.

- You will not be penalised for getting an answer wrong, even if you guess. A guess means that you have a 25% chance of getting the mark, so it is better to guess than to leave the question blank!

- If you really are unsure about a question, eliminate the obvious wrong answers and then make a calculated guess.

Four simple steps to answering Quantitative Reasoning questions

Step 1

Read the question carefully.

Step 2

Calculate your rough workings step-by-step using the whiteboard provided.

Step 3

Eliminate answers which are obviously incorrect from the five options.

Step 4

Mark the most accurate answer. (Remember to give your answer in the metric values as requested by the question.)

Quantitative Reasoning practice examples

Example 1

Company	Net Profit (£ million)	No of employees
Sharpe Buildings	123	23
Moben	123	12
Build Right	98	4
Home Essentials	23	13
Home Interiors	230	82

(handwritten annotations in Net Profit area: 5 3.17, 10.25, 24.5, 1.769, 2.8 04)

1   Which company made the most profit per employee?

    A   Sharpe Buildings

    B   Moben

    C   Build Right

    D   Home Essentials

    E   Home Interiors

2   If the company profits remain the same per employee for Moben, how many extra employees would the company have to employ to achieve an annual profit of £140 million? (Calculate your answer to the nearest whole number)

    A   2   *140 − 123 = 17*

    B   14   *17 ÷ 10.25 = 1.65*

    C   12

    D   13.65

    E   1.65

3   If Home Interiors' net profits increase by 10%, how much is the new
    total of the annual profit?

    A   £230,000

    B   £2,400,000,000

    C   £235,000,000

    D   £253,000,000

    E   £250,000,000

4   The following year, Home Essentials' profits decrease to £20 million.
    What is the percentage decrease? (Calculate your answer to the near-
    est whole number)

    A   3%

    B   13.04%

    C   13%

    D   13.1%

    E   14%

Example 2

Pie chart showing the number of staff at Global Insurance

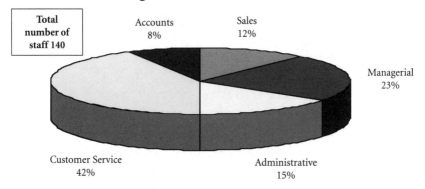

Total number of staff 140

Accounts 8%

Sales 12%

Managerial 23%

Customer Service 42%

Administrative 15%

5   What is the total number of staff in the Customer Service department? (Calculate your answer to the nearest whole number)

A   140

B   58

C   58.8

D   59

E   42

$140 \div 100 = 1.4$

$1.4 \times 42 = 58.8$

6   How many employees are there altogether in the Accounts and Sales
departments combined?

A   27

B   26

C   27.9

D   28

E   28.5

$1.4 \times 8 = 11.2$

$1.4 \times 12 = 16.8$

$11.2 + 16.8 = 28$

7   The Managerial department hires three more managers. Work out
    the new percentage of managers at Global Insurance. (Calculate your
    answer to one decimal place).

    A   24.5%

    B   24%

    C   24.47%

    D   24.4%

    E   24.57%

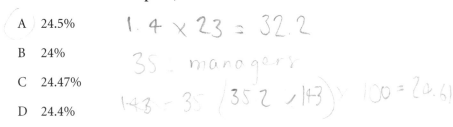

$1.4 \times 23 = 32.2$

35 managers

$143 - 35$ $(352 / 143) \times 100 = 24.61$

8   If 12 people are made redundant in the Customer Service depart-
    ment, how many staff members are there now in Customer Service?
    (Give your answer as a percentage to one decimal place)

    A   33.5%

    B   33.57%

    C   36%

    D   33%

    E   36.7%

$1.4 \times 42 = 58.8$

$59 - 12 = 47$

$170 - 12 = 138$

$(47 - 138) \times 100 = 34.05$

Example 3

Prices (£ Sterling)	Number of tickets to America (thousands)	
	2005	2006
0–129	12	89
130–149	34	987
150–159	12	123
160–169	129	12
170–179	23	24
180–189	5	56
190–199	32	43
200–209	123	12

9　How many tickets were sold in 2005 that were ≤ £169.00?

A　187

B　000129

C　187,000

D　129,000

E　129

10　What is the combined number of tickets ≥ £190.00 sold in 2005 and 2006?

A　210

B　21,000

C　210,000

D　2,101

E　3,210

11 **What is the mean number of tickets sold in each price range in 2006? (Give your answer as a whole number.)**

   A   168

   B   168,000

   C   168.25

   D   168.25000

   E   1,682,500

12 **By how much did the total number of tickets priced between £190 and £199 increase from 2005 to 2006? (Give your answer as a percentage to one decimal place.)**

   A   25%

   B   25.6%

   C   34.4%

   D   35.58%

   E   55.5%

Example 4

Colour of shoes	Number of shoes sold	Price of each shoe (£)
Red	121	12.90
Yellow	144	21.90
Brown	180	56.00
Black	121	67.00
White	234	12.90
Green	124	78.99
Pink	143	12.89
Grey	121	134.00

13 **Which colour of shoe generated the most income?**

A   Yellow

B   Green

C   White

D   Grey

E   Red

14 **What is the ratio of yellow to brown shoes sold?**

A   144:180

B   36:45

C   12:15

D   4:5

E   45:36

15 The red shoes were sold with a 56% discount. What is the new price? (Give your answer to two decimal places).

    A   £7.224

    B   £7.22

    C   £5.67

    D   £5.68

    E   £5.00

16 Which colour of shoe generated the least income?

    A   Red

    B   Pink

    C   White

    D   Black

    E   Yellow

Example 5

The bar graph below shows a candidate's scores on seven subtests. Each of the subtests are marked out of 50:

Candidate's test score on seven subtests

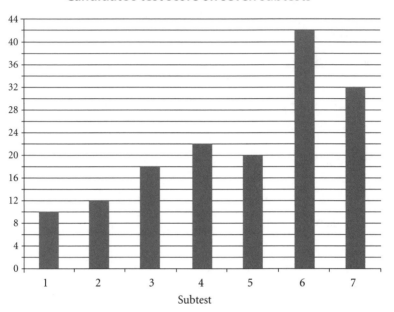

Subtest

17 **What is the mean of the candidate's test scores? (Calculate your answer to two decimal places.)**

A 22.285

B 22.29

C 22.28

D 22.2

E 22

18 What is the median of the candidate's test scores?

    A   20

    B   22

    C   22.29

    D   20.1

    E   21

19 What is the range of the test scores?

    A   42

    B   32

    C   20

    D   10

    E   22

20 What is the candidate's score on test 7 as a percentage?

    A   16%

    B   32%

    C   64%

    D   62%

    E   61%

Justifications of Quantitative Reasoning practice examples

Example 1

Question 1   Answer C

Step 1   The question is asking which company made the most profit per employee. In order to find this out we need to calculate the total net profit ÷ the number of employees per company. We calculate this for each company.

Sharpe Buildings = 123 ÷ 23 = 5.35 (to two decimal places)

Moben = 123 ÷ 12 = 10.25

Build Right = 98 ÷ 4 = 24.5

Home Essentials = 23 ÷ 13 = 1.77 (to two decimal places)

Home Interiors = 230 ÷ 82 = 2.80 (to two decimal places)

Step 2   We now compare the profits for each company per employee, which tells us that Build Right has the highest profit per employee.

Question 2   Answer A

Step 1   The company's profits for Moben are £123 million (net), £10.25 million per employee. (See above for the calculation of profit per employee).

Therefore each employee makes £10.25 million, from this we calculate how many employees would be needed to make £140 million.

We take the prospective profit, and divide this by the profit made per employee, which gives us the total employees needed to make a profit of £140 million.

140 ÷ 10.25 = 13.66 (to two decimal places)

= 14 (to the nearest whole number)

Step 2   The above calculation gives us the total number of employees to make a profit of £140 million. However we need to remember that there are already 12 employees working at the company. We simply need to work out the difference to find the extra number of employees needed.

14 – 12 = 2 (extra employees needed)

Question 3   Answer D

This question requires the calculation of a profit *increase*.

Step 1   We first need to calculate what 10% of Home Interiors' net profits are. We can work this out using the following calculation:

(Actual percentage ÷ 100) x total profit.

(10 ÷ 100) x 230 million = 23 million (10% of £230 million)

Step 2   We now add the total of the above calculation to the original profit.

230 million + 23 million = 253 million (new net profit total)

Question 4   Answer C

This question requires you to work out the actual percentage *decrease*.

The profits have dropped from 230 million to 200 million – this is a decrease of 30 million.

Step 1   We need to work out the decrease as a percentage; we calculate this by dividing the actual decrease by the original total and multiplying the sum by 100.

(30 million ÷ 230 million) x 100 = 13.04 (to 2 decimal places)

= 13 (to the nearest whole number)

Question 5   Answer D

We are given the total number of staff there (140); 42% of 140 staff members are part of the Customer Service department. Taking these values into account, we now need to work out the actual number of staff (in Customer Service) as a whole number. We use the following calculation:

(Percentage of staff in Customer Service department ÷ 100) x Total number of staff.

(42 ÷ 100) x 140 = 58.8

= 59 (to the nearest whole number).

Question 6   Answer D

Step 1

Using the above formula, we need to work out the number of staff in the Accounts and Sales departments. As above we are already given the percentage of staff in both sectors. 8% of 140 members of staff are in the Accounts sector and 12% are in the Sales sector.

(8 ÷ 100) x 140 = 11.2 (members of staff in Accounts)

= 11 (to the nearest whole number)

(12 ÷ 100) x 140 = 16.8 (members of staff in Sales)

 = 17 (to the nearest whole number)

* When working out totals of staff members it is important to take note that staff members cannot be represented as decimal points, therefore it is wiser to use whole numbers.

Step 2

We now add the two totals up and calculate the total number of staff in Accounts and Sales.

11+ 17 = 28

Question 7   **Answer A**

23% of 140 staff members are Managers. Three more members have now joined.

Step 1   We first need to find out how many staff members are equal to 23%.

Therefore, using the same calculations as in Questions 5 and 6:

(Percentage of staff in customer service department ÷ 100) x Total number of staff.

(23 ÷ 100) x 140 = 32.2 (members of staff who are Managers)

= 32 (to the nearest whole number)

Step 2   We now add the three new members of staff to the original staff total in the Managerial sector.

3 + 32 = 35 (new total members of staff in the managerial sector)

Step 3   Now we calculate the above total as a percentage. (Remember to add the extra three members of staff to the final total members of staff in the company.)

(35 ÷ 143) x 100 = 24.47

= **24.5% (to one decimal place)**

Question 8   **Answer E**

Step 1   We first calculate how many members of staff there are in the Customer Service department. We only know that 42% of 140 members are in the Customer Service department.

We can find out the number of staff by using the following calculation:

(Percentage of staff in sector ÷ 100) x total number of staff in the company

42 ÷ 100 x 140 = 58.8 (59 members of staff to the nearest whole number).

Step 2   We now need to subtract the total number of staff who are
                 made redundant from the above total.

                 59 – 12 = 47 members of staff are leftover

Step 3   We then need to calculate 47 staff members out of 128 (as
                 12 people have left, therefore the total of the staff mem-
                 bers in the organisation also decrease) as a percentage.

                 (47 ÷ 128) x 100 = 36.7% (to 1 decimal place).

Question 9   **Answer C**

                 We need to calculate how many tickets sold in 2005 which
                 cost equal to or less than (≤) £169.00

                 Therefore we add up the amount from each price range
                 below £169.00.

                 12 + 34 + 12 + 129 = 187.

                 **The numbers of tickets are shown in the table as thou-
                 sands, therefore the answer is 187,000.**

Question 10   **Answer C**

                 We need to calculate how many tickets sold in 2005 and
                 2006 which cost equal to or more than (≥) £190.00

                 Therefore we add up the amount from each price range
                 (from 2005 and 2006) > £190.00

                 32 + 123 (in 2005) =155

                 43 +12 (in 2006) = 55

                 155 + 55 = 210

                 **The numbers of tickets are shown in the table as thou-
                 sands, therefore the answer is 210,000**

Question 11   Answer B

The question is asking you to calculate the mean number or the average number of tickets sold within each price range in 2006.

Therefore we add up how many tickets there are divided by the 8 categories.

(89 + 987 + 123 + 12 + 24 + 56 + 43 + 12) ÷ 8 = 168.25

= 168,000 (to the nearest thousand)

Question 12   Answer C

In 2005, 32,000 tickets were sold between the prices of £190.00 and £199.00

In 2006, 43,000 tickets were sold between the prices of £190.00 and £199.00

Step 1   We first find out the difference of the two totals:

43,000 – 32,000 = 11,000

Therefore in 2006 ticket sales increased by 11,000.

Step 2   We now need to work out the above total as a percentage (working in thousands):

(11,000 ÷ 32,000) x 100 = 34.4% (to one decimal place).

Question 13   Answer D

Step 1   We need to calculate the total income generated on each different shoe. (Tip: you do not need to work out the total income generated for those not listed in the answer options – this way you are able to save more time).

We work out the income generated by multiplying the total number of shoes sold by the price of one shoe.

Yellow   144 x £21.90 = £3,153.60

Green   124 x £78.99 = £9,794.76

White   234 x £12.90 = £3,018.60

Grey   **121 x £134.00 = £16,214**

Red   121 x £12.90 = £1,560.90

Therefore the grey coloured shoes generated the greatest income.

Question 14   Answer D

There are 144 yellow shoes to 180 brown shoes. This can be written as 144:180

We can then reduce this ratio by dividing each side by 12 = 12:15

The above total can be reduced even further by dividing the answer by 3 = **4:5**

Therefore for every 4 yellow shoes there are 5 brown shoes.

Question 15   Answer D

The original price of one pair of red shoes is £12.90. We need to find 56% of this total.

Step 1   We calculate 56% of £12.90 as follows: (56 ÷ 100) x £12.90 = £7.224

Step 2   We then subtract the above total from the original price:

£12.90 − £7.224 = £5.676

= **£5.68** (to two decimal places)

Question 16   Answer A

We already have the total income generated from some of the answer choices (see Question 13)

Yellow 144 x £21.90 = £3,153.6

White 234 x £12.90 = £3,018.6

Red   121 x £12.90 = £1,560.9

However we still need to calculate the income generated for the pink and black shoes.

Pink   143 x £12.89 = £1,843.27

Black   121 x £67.00 = £8,107

The red shoes generated the least income.

Question 17   Answer B

We need to find out the candidate's mean/average score amongst the subtests. We can calculate this by adding up the results across all the subtests and dividing this by the total number of subtests.

(10 + 12 + 18 + 22 + 20 + 42 + 32) ÷ 7 = 22.29 (to 2 decimal places).

Question 18   Answer A

To calculate the median of the test scores we need to distribute each test score in ascending order and then find the middle value.

10, 12, 18, **20,** 22, 32, 42

20 is therefore the median of the candidate's scores.

Question 19   Answer B

To calculate the range of the test scores, we need to subtract the highest value from the lowest value.

42 – 10 = 32 (range of scores)

Question 20   Answer C

The candidate scored 32 out of 50 possible marks on subtest 7. We are able to calculate the percentage by dividing the raw score by the total number of possible marks; we then multiply the total by 100.

(32 ÷ 50) x 100 = 64%

Chapter 5

The Abstract Reasoning Subtest

This section of the UKCAT explores a candidate's ability to infer relationships using divergent and convergent thinking. This specific type of test will explore your ability to solve abstract logical problems and requires no prior knowledge or educational experience. As such, these specific tests are the least affected by the candidate's educational experience, and high performance in this subtest is arguably the best indication of pure intelligence or innate reasoning ability.

Divergent thinking encompasses the ability to generate many different ideas about a topic in a short period of time. Convergent thinking is related to reasoning that combines information focusing on solving a problem (especially solving problems that have a single correct solution). Convergent thinking involves combining or joining different ideas together based on common elements.

Achieving high scores in the Abstract Reasoning subtest reflects a candidate's ability to process multiple visual images and identify patterns and relationships between the information provided, which is an essential skill required of a healthcare professional.

Abstract Reasoning tests are usually presented in sequences and patterns, which involve symbols and shapes.

When attempting such questions, we need to understand the following concepts:

- Symmetry – are the shapes in a symmetrical format?

- Number patterns – is there a common pattern in the sequence of numbers, e.g. 2, 4, 6, 8 and so on?

- Size – do the shapes vary in size?

- Shapes – are there specific shapes being used?

- Characteristics – are the symbols and shapes curved; do they have straight lines or angles?

- Rotation – are the shapes or symbols rotated clockwise or anti-clockwise?

- Direction – are the symbols or shapes in any specific direction, i.e. are they aligned diagonally, horizontally or vertically?

- Lines – are they continuous or dashed?

The Abstract Reasoning subtest consists of 13 stems. Each stem comprises two sets (Set A and Set B) which each contain six shape formations. You will then be presented with five further shape options which are the lead-in questions. You will be expected to identify whether each lead-in question belongs to either 'Set A', 'Set B' or 'Neither'.

You will be allocated a time limit of 16 minutes for the Abstract Reasoning subtest which equates to approximately 15 seconds for each answer. This time allocation includes one minute for administration purposes.

Summary of Abstract Reasoning structure

Stem

The stem will consist of a pair of shapes known as 'Set A' and 'Set B.' Each set will contain a total of six shapes, all of which will have common themes. There will be a total of 13 stems.

Lead-in question

For each stem there will be a total of five shapes which act as the lead-in questions. There will be a total of 65 lead-in questions.

Choices

Your task will be to decide whether the test shapes are part of 'Set A' or 'Set B' or 'Neither'.

Only one of the choices will be correct.

Time limit = 16 minutes. Therefore you will have approximately 15 seconds per question

When you are working through the UKCAT subtests it can be counter-productive to monitor exactly how long you spend on answering each question, especially when you need to read through and digest the information presented in the stem. Therefore a more useful time management approach is to divide each subtest into four quarters. So, in the case of the Abstract Reasoning subtest, after approximately four minutes you should be working on the fourth stem, after approximately eight minutes you should be commencing the seventh stem and so on. If you find yourself falling behind at these points you know that you need to pick up the pace.

Example of an Abstract Reasoning question

Set A   Set B

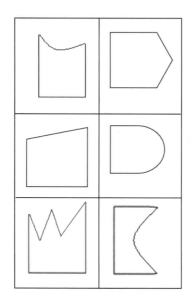 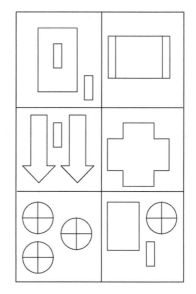

Test shape 1

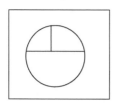

Answer: Set A, Set B, or Neither

Abstract Reasoning hints and tips

Throughout the Abstract Reasoning subtest the shapes can be ordered in a variety of ways. The various patterns that can be used to distinguish between the shapes include:

- Symmetry – are the shapes symmetrical?

- Number patterns – is there a common pattern in the sequence of numbers, e.g. 2, 4, 6, 8 and so on?

- Size – do the shapes vary in size?

- Shapes – are there specific shapes being used?

- Characteristics – are the symbols and shapes curved; do they possess straight lines or angles?

- Rotation – are the shapes or symbols rotated clockwise or anti-clockwise?

- Direction – are the symbols or shapes in any specific direction i.e. are they aligned diagonally, horizontally or vertically?

- Lines of shapes – are they continuous, dashed or double lines?

Symmetrical Characteristics

- Some of the larger symmetrical shapes may be replicated amongst smaller '*distracter*' shapes.

- Some shapes may seem symmetrical at first glance but are in fact asymmetrical, such as a parallelogram.

- Some sets contain shapes which are symmetrical and are only made up of straight lines while asymmetrical shapes may be curved or vice versa.

- Some symmetrical shapes may have a dotted or dashed outline, asymmetrical shapes may have a solid outline or vice versa.

- Some sets may have symmetrical shapes which are shaded in black, while asymmetrical shapes may be white or vice versa.

Number patterns

- Certain number patterns may be symbolised by specific shapes. For example, if a set contained shapes in sets of 2, 4 and 6 they may be represented by small triangles.

- Some number patterns are often replicated in both sets; however the accommodating shapes may differ from one set to another. For example, in Set A, if there are small triangles in groups of 2, 4 and 6 and small circles in groups of 3, 6 and 9, this pattern may be reversed in Set B whereby there will be small circles in groups of 2, 4 and 6 and small triangles in groups of 3, 6 and 9.

- Some number patterns may be represented with various types of shading, e.g. black or white shading or different outlines e.g. dotted, dashed or solid outlines.

Size

- Do the shapes vary in size?

- Are certain sized shapes positioned in specific areas in a set?

- Often the same sized shapes are used in both sets, although they are positioned differently.

  For example in Set A, there could be three different sized circular shapes – small, medium and large. The smallest shape could always be positioned within the largest shape. The same sized shapes may also be used in Set B, however the rules change slightly and instead the medium sized circular shape could be positioned within the largest shape.

- Shapes may be shaded or unshaded, for example curved shapes are shaded in black and shapes with straight lines are left white.

Characteristics

- Some sets may contain curved or straight lined shapes.

- A common method of causing confusion is to combine a mixture of curved and straight lines within a shape.

- Other sets may contain shapes which possess a dashed or solid outline or even a mixture of both.

- Some shapes may be present in differing quantities.

Rotation and direction

- Shapes can be positioned horizontally or vertically, and towards the middle, top, bottom, right or left of the test box.

- Shapes can be positioned in either a clockwise or anti-clockwise position.

Three simple steps to Abstract Reasoning

Once you acknowledge the various ways in which the shapes can be presented, you will find it easier to apply this knowledge if you follow the three simple steps below:

Step 1

First identify the different shapes and symbols used within each stem. Look for characteristics such as size, number and colour.

Step 2

Try to identify any patterns which the shapes or symbols form, such as reoccurring number patterns, rotation and positioning of shapes, symmetry and direction of shapes.

Step 3

Try to identify the next part of the sequence for each lead-in question, and relate them to either 'Set A', 'Set B' or 'Neither'. If you really are unsure of the answer go with your gut instinct rather than leaving a blank.

Below you will find some examples of the types of Abstract Reasoning questions you will face when you attempt the UKCAT.

Abstract Reasoning Practice Examples

Example 1

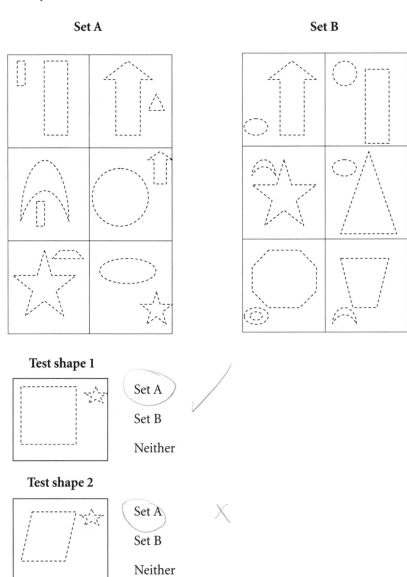

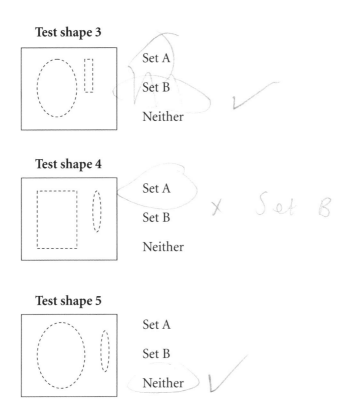

Test shape 3

Set A

Set B

Neither

Test shape 4

Set A

Set B

Neither

$\times$ Set B

Test shape 5

Set A

Set B

Neither

Example 2

Set A

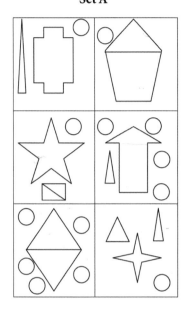

Set B

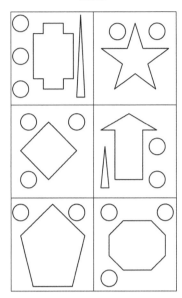

Test shape 1

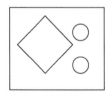

Set A

Set B

Neither

X Set B

Test shape 2

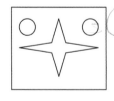

Set A

Set B

Neither

X Set B

Test shape 3

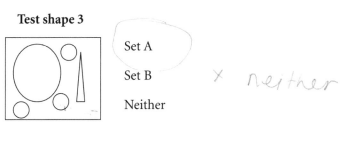

Set A

Set B   ✗   neither

Neither

Test shape 4

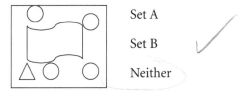

Set A

Set B   ✓

Neither

Test shape 5

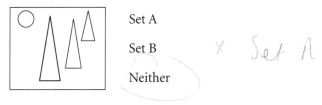

Set A

Set B   ✗   Set A

Neither

Example 3

Set A

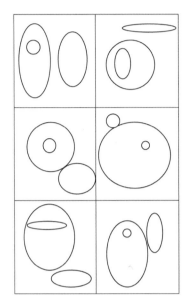

Set B

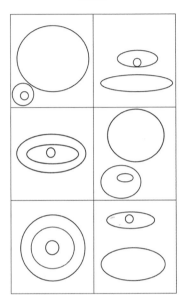

Test shape 1

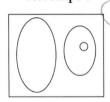

Set A

Set B   ✗   Set B

Neither

Test shape 2

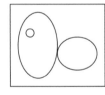

Set A   ✗   Set A

Set B

Neither

Test shape 3

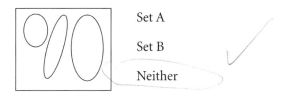

Set A

Set B

Neither

Test shape 4

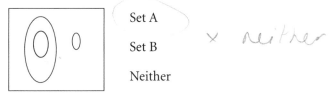

Set A

Set B

Neither

✗ neither

Test shape 5

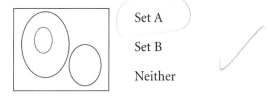

Set A

Set B

Neither

Example 4

Set A

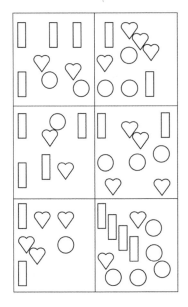

Set B

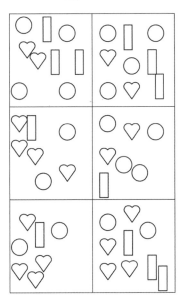

Test shape 1

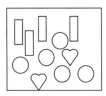

Set A

Set B

Neither

Test shape 2

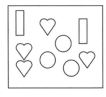

Set A

Set B

Neither

Test shape 3

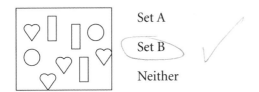

Set A

Set B

Neither

Test shape 4

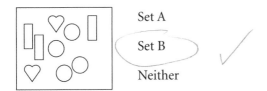

Set A

Set B

Neither

Test shape 5

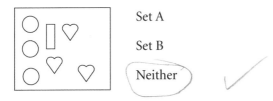

Set A

Set B

Neither

Example 5

Set A	Set B

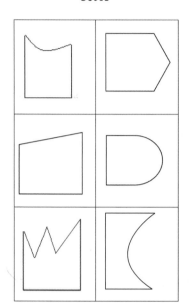

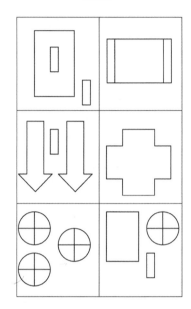

Test shape 1

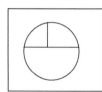

Set A

(Set B) × Set A

Neither

Test shape 2

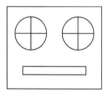

Set A

Set B ✓

Neither

Test shape 3

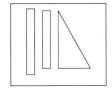

Set A

Set B

Neither

✓

Test shape 4

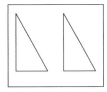

Set A

Set B

Neither

✗ Set A

Test shape 5

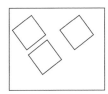

Set A

Set B

Neither

✗ Set B

Example 6

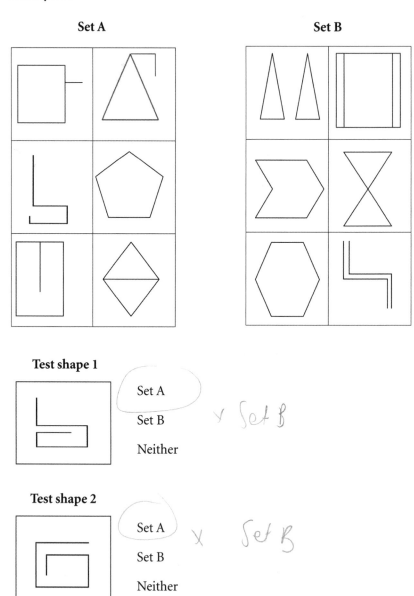

Set A

Set B

Test shape 1

Set A

Set B   ✗ Set B

Neither

Test shape 2

Set A   ✗ Set B

Set B

Neither

Test shape 3

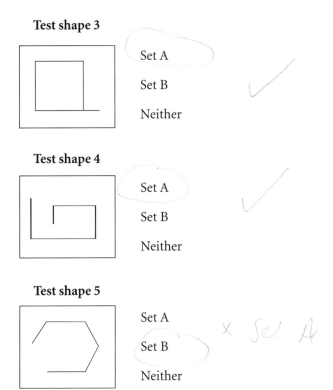

Set A

Set B   ✓

Neither

Test shape 4

Set A   ✓

Set B

Neither

Test shape 5

Set A

Set B   ✗ Set A

Neither

Example 7

Set A

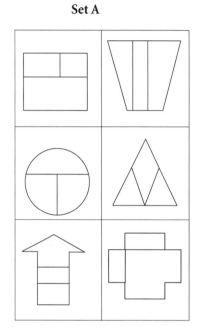

Set B

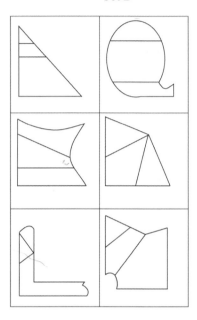

Test shape 1

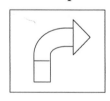

Set A

Set B ⊗ ✗ neither

Neither

Test shape 2

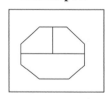

Set A

Set B

Neither

✓

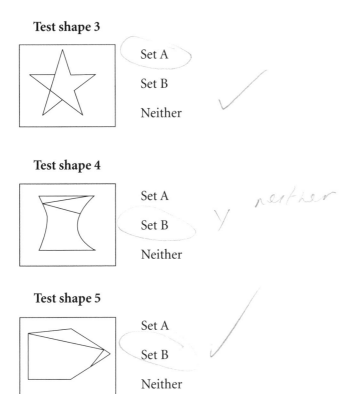

Test shape 3

Set A

Set B

Neither ✓

Test shape 4

Set A

Set B   y   neither

Neither

Test shape 5

Set A ✓

Set B

Neither

Justifications of Abstract Reasoning Practice Questions

Example 1

Set A

In this set there are large straight and curved symmetrical shapes. The main rule for this set is that each shape must have a smaller corresponding symmetrical shape which is made of straight lines only.

Set B

In this set there are large symmetrical shapes made only from straight lines. The main rule for this set is that each shape must have a smaller corresponding symmetrical shape which is made of curved lines only.

Test shape 1   Answer: Set A

The smaller shape is made of straight lines, and for this reason it belongs to set A. It cannot be related to set B as the smaller shape would have to be of a curved nature.

Test shape 2   Answer: Neither set

The large shape is not symmetrical; therefore it cannot belong to either set.

Test shape 3   Answer: Set A

The smaller shape is made of straight lines, and therefore belongs to set A. It cannot belong to set B for two reasons; first, the smaller shape would need to be made of curved lines and secondly, the large shape can only be made of straight lines.

Test shape 4   Answer: Set B

The smaller shape is curved and hence belongs to set B.

Test shape 5   Answer: Neither set

The smaller shape is curved, which is a characteristic of set B; however the test shape cannot belong to set B as the large shape is also curved and this set only has large shapes made of straight lines.

Example 2

Set A

In this set there are large symmetrical shapes made from straight lines only. The main rule in this set is that in each shape there must be at least one or more triangular shapes, either within shapes or outside shapes. The white circles are used as distracters.

Set B

In this set there are large symmetrical shapes which are made from straight lines only. In this set the circles are in pairs or threes and the triangles are used as distracters.

Test shape 1   Answer: Set B

The test shape belongs to set B, as the circles are presented in a pair. As well as this, the large shape is made of straight lines. The test shape cannot belong to set A, as there are no corresponding triangles.

Test shape 2   Answer: Set B

The explanation is the same as above.

Test shape 3   Answer: Neither set

The test shape does not belong to either group as the large shape is curved. Both sets have the characteristic of having one large shape which is made up of straight lines only.

Test shape 4   Answer: Neither set

The large shape is not symmetrical and this is a requirement of both sets.

Test shape 5   Answer: Set A

There are three triangles which are a requirement of set A; the test shape cannot be related to set B as there is only one circle instead of two or three.

Example 3

Set A

In this set there should only be three circular shapes, which are of three different sizes: small, medium and large. The smallest shape should always be within the largest shape.

Set B

In a similar way to set A, there should only be three circular shapes, which are of three different sizes: small, medium and large. The only difference is the position of the smallest shape which should be placed with the medium sized circular shape.

Test shape 1   Answer: Set B

The test shape belongs to set B, as the smallest shape is within the medium sized shape. The test shape cannot belong to set A, as the smallest shape would need to be within the largest shape.

Test shape 2   Answer: Set A

The test shape belongs to set A as the smallest shape is within the largest shape. The test shape cannot belong to set B, as the smallest shape would need to be within the medium sized shape.

Test shape 3   Answer: Neither set

The smallest circular shape is not within the largest or the medium shape, therefore it does not follow the rules of either set.

Test shape 4   Answer: Neither set

As above, the smallest shape is not within any shape, and again does not follow the rules for either set.

Test shape 5   Answer: Set A

The test shape belongs to set A as the smallest shape is within the largest shape. The test shape cannot belong to set B, as the smallest shape would need to be within the medium sized shape

Example 4

Set A

In this set there are small rectangles, hearts and circles. The rules for this set are as follows:

- For every 4 rectangles there should be 2 corresponding hearts.
- For every 2 rectangles there should be 4 corresponding hearts.
- The circles are used as distracters.

Set B

As above, the set contains small rectangles, hearts and circles. The rules for this set are as follows:

- For every 4 circles there should be 2 corresponding hearts.
- For every 2 circles there should be 4 corresponding hearts.
- The rectangles are used as distracters.

Test shape 1   Answer: Set A

In this test shape there are 4 rectangles to 2 corresponding hearts. The test shape cannot belong to set B, as there are 5 circles instead of 4 circles to 2 hearts.

Test shape 2   Answer: Set A

The test shape contains 2 rectangles to 4 corresponding hearts, which are characteristics of set A. The test shape cannot be part of set B, as there are 3 circles instead of 2 circles to 4 hearts.

Test shape 3   Answer: Set B

There are 4 hearts to 2 circles, which are characteristics of set B. The test shape cannot be part of set A as there are 3 rectangles instead of 2 rectangles to 4 hearts.

Test shape 4   Answer: Set B

In this set there are 4 circles to 2 hearts which therefore means they are part of set B. They cannot be part of set A as there are 3 rectangles instead of 4 rectangles to 2 hearts.

Test shape 5   Answer: Neither set

None of the shapes correspond to the number patterns in either set.

Example 5

Set A

In this set there are symmetrical and non-symmetrical shapes, which are made up of straight and curved lines. Each of the test shapes must only have 2 right angles.

Set B

There are various symmetrical shapes, consisting of both straight and curved lines. The rule in this set is that there must be a total of 12 external and/or internal right angles only.

Test shape 1   Answer: Set A

The test shape has a total of 2 right angles and hence belongs to set A. The test shape cannot belong to set B as there are not enough right angles

Test shape 2   Answer: Set B

The test shape has a total of 12 right angles and therefore belongs to set B. The test shape cannot be part of set A as there are too many right angles.

Test shape 3   Answer: Neither set

There are a total of 9 right angles and for this reason the test shape does not belong to either group.

Test shape 4   Answer: Set A

The test shape has a total of 2 right angles and hence belongs to set A. The test shape cannot belong to set B as there are not enough right angles

Test shape 5   Answer: Set B

The test shape has as total of 12 right angles and therefore belongs to set B. The test shape cannot be part of set A as there are too many right angles.

Example 6

Set A
The set consists of any shape(s) made out of only 5 lines.

Set B
The set consists of any shape(s) made out of only 6 lines.

Test shape 1   Answer: Set B
The test shape is made out of 6 lines.

Test shape 2   Answer: Set B
The test shape is made out of 6 lines.

Test shape 3   Answer: Set A
The test shape is made out of 5 lines.

Test shape 4   Answer: Set A
The test shape is made out of 5 lines.

Test shape 5   Answer: Set A
The test shape is made out of 5 lines.

Example 7

Set A

The set contains straight and curved symmetrical shapes, which have been divided into 3 parts.

Set B

The set contains straight and curved non-symmetrical shapes. Again, each shape has been divided into 3 parts. The main rule is that each shape must have only 1 right angle.

Test shape 1　　Answer: Neither set

The test shape is not symmetrical and therefore cannot belong to set A. The test shape also cannot belong to set B as there are 7 right angles instead of one.

Test shape 2　　Answer: Set A

The test shape belongs to set A, as it is symmetrical and is divided into to 3 parts. The test shape cannot belong to set B, as there are 8 right angles instead of one.

Test shape 3　　Answer: Set A

This test shape is symmetrical, and is divided into 3 parts.

Test shape 4　　Answer: Neither set

The test shape is not symmetrical and therefore cannot belong to set A. The test shape also cannot belong to set B as there no right angles.

Test shape 5　　Answer: Set B

The test shape belongs to set B, as it is divided into 3 parts and includes 1 right angle. The test shape cannot belong to set A as the shape is not symmetrical.

Chapter 6

The Decision Analysis Subtest

The Decision Analysis test measures a candidate's ability to translate and make sense of coded information. This type of test measures a candidate's quality of decision making in terms of accuracy, adequacy and the time taken in which the decision is made. Individuals must possess an exceptional ability to translate and identify related information, separate facts from fiction and consider all issues they are presented with. Achieving a high score in the Decision Analysis subtest reflects a candidate's ability to make decisions in real-life situations where the information provided is complex and from various sources.

The UKCAT Decision Analysis subtest consists of one scenario and 26 related items which form the basis of questions asked. The scenario itself may contain a table, text and various other sources of information and codes. You will be requested to interpret information given in the questions using the facts provided in the scenario.

You will find at times that the information which you have is either incomplete or that it does not make sense. You will then need to make your best judgement based on the codes, rather than what you expect to see or what you think is reasonable. **Ensure that you base your decisions solely on the information provided to you.** There will always be a best answer which makes the most sense based on all the information presented. It is important that you understand that this test is based on judgements rather than simply applying rules and logic.

The Decision Analysis subtest differs from the other UKCAT subtests in that there can be more than five answer options for each question. Another notable difference from the other subtests is that candidates may be asked to give more than one response for a particular question. However, if this is the case then this will always be clearly stated within the question. You will have a time limit of 30 minutes for this section, which includes one minute for administration purposes, to answer 26 questions equating to just over one minute per question.

Summary of Decision Analysis structure

Stem

In this subtest you will be presented with one scenario comprising various facts and information, including codes.

Lead-in question

There will be 26 individual lead-in questions, based on just the one scenario (the stem).

Choices

For each of the lead-in questions you will be given a choice of five or more answers. These will be represented as A, B, C, D or E etc. In the previous subtests there was always only one correct answer. In this subtest you may be given the option of choosing more than one correct answer. This will always be clearly indicated in the lead-in question.

Time limit = 30 minutes. Therefore you will have 69 seconds per question.

When you are working through the UKCAT subtests it can be counter-productive to monitor exactly how long you spend on answering each question, especially when you need to read through and digest the information presented in the stem. Therefore a more useful time management approach is to divide each subtest into four quarters. So, in the case of the Decision Analysis subtest, after approximately seven and half minutes you should be working on the seventh question, after approximately 13 minutes you should be commencing the fourteenth question and so on. If you find yourself falling behind at these points you know that you need to pick up the pace.

Example of Decision Analysis question

Scenario (Stem)

A group of historians have discovered a cave with various paintings and symbols on the walls. The team have managed to decode some of the messages; these are presented in the table below. Your task is to examine particular codes or sentences and then choose the best interpretation of the code from one of five possible choices.

You will find, at times, that the information which you have is either incomplete or does not make sense. You will need to make your best judgement based on the codes rather than what you expect to see or what you think is reasonable. There will always be a best answer which makes the most sense based on all of the information presented. It is important that you understand that this test is based on judgements rather than simply applying rules and logic.

Operating Codes	Routine Codes	Specialist Codes
A = Opposite	1 = Sun	♓ = Happy
B = Decrease	2 = People	❑ = Angry
C = Negative	3 = Building	◆ = Shy
D = Cold	4 = City	♒ = Assertive
E = Similar	5 = Yesterday	● = Intelligent
F = Disregard	6 = Run	○ = Extraverted
G = Quickly	7 = Sand	♐ = Daring
H = Merge	8 = Danger	♋ = Trusting
I = Up	9 = Tonight	⌘ = Unstable
J = Weak	10 = Water	
K = Hard	11 = Tomorrow	
L = Desire	12 = Lonely	
	13 = Ice	
	14 = Sea	
	15 = Footprints	
	16 = Storm	
	17 = Light	
	18 = Anatomy	
	19 = He	
	20 = Structure	
	21 = Security	
	22 = Natural	
	23 = They	
	24 = Colour	
	25 = Breeze	
	26 = Thought	

Question 1

[handwritten: Sad no people run building]

Examine the following coded message: (A, ⊁), (A, 2), (6, 3)

Now examine the following sentences and try to determine the most likely interpretation of the code.

A   The building made people happy

B   I felt sad so I scampered home

C   Happy people scampered towards the building

D   I feel sad inside the building

E   People in the building were happy

Decision Analysis hints and tips

The following are common mistakes to look for when interpreting codes in a Decision Analysis subtest:

- **Various interpretations** of the same word can be used, e.g. 'present', which could refer to time, as in 'the present moment', or otherwise to a gift, as in 'a birthday present'.

- Some of the answer options may include all of the encoded words but may not make logical or grammatical sense.

- Some answer options **may not include all of the interpreted code words.**

- The interpreted words are **not necessarily in a specific order.** Therefore do not make the mistake of necessarily interpreting the codes in the exact order they are presented.

- **Do not spend too long on a difficult question.** Difficult questions are often easily identifiable by the length and complexity of the code – effective time management is key.

- Words within brackets are usually combined to give one meaning and should not be used as separate words within answer options.

- Certain codes require you to give your answer in a specific tense such as 'past', 'present' or 'future'. These answers do not require you to actually state the word unless specified by other codes.

- Base your answer on the information provided – do not make subjective judgements.

- Where you are unable to distinguish between two answer options go with your gut feeling as this is normally correct.

- As you work through each question use your whiteboard to make a note of the code interpretations, to avoid confusion.

- You may be asked a question where you are provided with a line of text that you must convert into the correct code sequence.

Three simple steps to interpreting Decision Analysis questions

Step 1

Interpret the coded information given in the lead-in question and write the words down on your whiteboard – remember to pay special attention to words in brackets.

Step 2

Translate the meaning of combined codes where applicable.

Step 3

Relate the words to each of the answer options; remember to take the following into account:

- Do the answer options make use of all of the words within the code?

- Which of the answer options are clearly incorrect or contain information not referred to in the scenario, and are therefore easy to eliminate?

- Dotheansweroptionsmakeuseofthecombinedwordsandwordsinbrackets correctly?

- Is the answer given in an order that reflects the code correctly and makes sense?

- Which answer options are clearly correct, and of these, which potential correct answer options arrive at the best interpretation of the code?

- An answer can still be correct if it does not contain the exact interpretation but is the best fit of all the answer options provided.

Decision Analysis practice example questions

Scenario One

A group of archaeologists have discovered a hidden pyramid. They have found hieroglyphics on the walls which show various codes. The team have managed to decode some of the messages; these are presented in figure 1 below. Your task is to examine particular codes or sentences and then choose the best interpretation of the code from one of five possible choices.

You will find that, at times, the information you have is either incomplete or does not make sense. You will then need to make your best judgement based on the codes rather than what you expect to see or what you think is reasonable. There will always be a best answer which makes the most sense based on all the information presented. It is important that you understand that this test is based on judgements rather than simply applying rules and logic.

Figure 1:

Operating codes	Routine codes
1 = Opposite	A = Sprint
2 = Positive	B = Night
3 = Together	C = Apparatus
4 = Single	D = Public
5 = Different	E = Shade
6 = Challenging	F = Crash
7 = Enjoyable	G = Structure
8 = Prefer	H = Number
9 = Closed	I = Word
10 = Increased	J = Individual
11 = Past	K = Liquid
12 = Future	L = Oxygen
13 = Present	M = He
14 = Plural	N = Human
15 = Conditional	O = Achievement
16 = Repeated	P = Harm
17 = Alter	Q = Body
	R = Tremor
	S = Building
	T = Fire
	U = Senses
	V = Disaster
	W = Take
	X = Part
	Y = Cold

Apparatus oxygen senses (increased fire)

Example 1

Examine the following coded message: **C, L, U, (10,T)**

Now examine the following sentences and try to determine the most likely interpretation of the code.

A   The Bunsen burner smelt of gas and was very hot.

B   The apparatus was very hot as the air increased.   *A*

C   The fireplace had a large amount of air in the pipes.

D   You could smell the gas from the fire.

E   The fireplace smelt of gas.

Example 2

(opposite take) human crash she present

Examine the following coded message: **(1, W), N, F, (1, M), 13**

Now examine the following sentences and try to determine the most likely interpretation of the code.

A   She took the human out of the crash.

B   He pulled himself out of the crash.

C   She is only human.

D   She was only human after she came out of the crash.

E   She gave the crushed human the kiss of life.

Example 3

Shade day fire past

Examine the following coded message: **E, (1, B), T, 11**

Now examine the following sentences and try to determine the most likely interpretation of the code.

A   The night gave shade from the heat.

B   The red fire happened in the day.

C   There was no shade in the heat of the day.

D   The shade gave no protection from the fire.

E   It was a red hot day.

Example 4

Examine the following coded message: **10, K, L, B, (1, B), 12**

Now examine the following sentences and try to determine the most likely interpretation of the code.

A   It was very wet at night, more so than the day.

B   It rained a lot today, and will be drier at night.

C   It was very wet tonight.

D   The liquid increased today, and dried at night.

E   The air was very dry as it had been raining today.

increased liquid oxygen night

day

(opposite night) future.

Example 5   conditional future (liquid increase) structure

Examine the following coded message: **15, 12, (K, 10), G, F**

Now examine the following sentences and try to determine the two most likely interpretations of the code.   crash

A   The bridge is flooded heavily.

B   Rain water flooded the structure and offices.

C   The bridge will fall in the evening.

D   If the water level increases the bridge will crash.

E   There is a lot of water under the building.

Jack was 'ere 2012

Example 6

Examine the following coded message: (14, H), 6, M, (14, B, 10), O, 13

Now examine the following sentences and try to determine the most likely interpretation of the code.

A   He made the number of words challenging.

B   He finds Maths and English examinations very difficult.

C   He makes the number of words increasingly difficult.

D   He made the number of words increasingly challenging.

E   The number of words was increasingly difficult.

(plural number) challenging he
(plural word) increased achievement
present

Example 7

Examine the following coded message: **(14, M), U, 11, F, V, (1, B)**

Now examine the following sentences and try to determine the two most likely interpretations of the code.

A   The men would have seen the catastrophe, as the crash had occurred in the day.

B   He could sense the danger, on the condition that there was daylight.

C   The men could see the disasters had struck at night, as soon as they heard the crash.

D   The crash was a catastrophe, the men could have seen more in the daylight.

E   Crashes caused by men have been absolute disasters.

(Plural he) Senses past

crash disaster (opposite night day)

Further codes have been added which are under the heading of emotions

Figure 2:

Operating codes	Routine codes	Emotions
1 = Opposite	A = Sprint	✳ = Excited
2 = Positive	B = Night	∝ = Worried
3 = Together	C = Apparatus	༡ = Afraid
4 = Single	D = Public	⊰ = Happy
5 = Different	E = Shade	⊗ = Nervous
6 = Challenging	F = Crash	☻ = Sad
7 = Enjoyable	G = Structure	= Surprised
8 = Prefer	H = Number	♎ = Angry
9 = Closed	I = Word	
10 = Increased	J = Individual	
11 = Past	K = Liquid	
12 = Future	L = Oxygen	
13 = Present	M = He	
14 = Plural	N = Human	
15 = Conditional	O = Achievement	
16 = Repeated	P = Harm	
17 = Alter	Q = Body	
	R = Tremor	
	S = Building	
	T = Fire	
	U = Senses	
	V = Disaster	
	W =Take	
	X = Part	
	Y = Cold	
	Z = Hazard	

Increased past (opposite he)
acheivement take happ

Example 8

Examine the following coded message: **10, 11, (1, M), O, W, ✂**

Now examine the following sentences and try to determine the most likely interpretation of the code.

A She is achieving a lot and is very happy.

B He was very happy when he received his exam results.

C She was very content when she received her exam results.

D She is very happy with her exam results.

E She was very unhappy when she received her exam results.

Example 9

Examine the following coded message: **(X, Q), (1, M), U, (T, V, K) 13, R**

Now examine the following sentences and try to determine the most likely interpretation of the code.

A The womens' bodies trembled as they heard the fire.

B Her body was shaking, as she heard the thunder.

C Her body shook as she read about the volcano.

D Her hands trembled with fear as she saw the volcano erupt.

E Her hands are shaking as she sees the volcano erupt.

(part body) (she) senses
(fire disaster liquid) present
tremor

Example 10

[handwritten: acheivement (op negative)]
[handwritten: sad/surprised shade) (opposite he)]

Examine the following coded message: **O, (1, 2), (●, E), (1, M)**

Now examine the following sentences and try to determine the most likely interpretation of the code.

A   He felt blue as he did not pass his exams.

B   She felt sad, as the shade was not achievable.

C   She felt sad like the shade of blue.

D   She felt blue as she did not pass her course.

E   She felt sad as she did not achieve her shade.

[handwritten: conditional present individual]

Example 11

[handwritten: (plural word) (opposite positive)]

Examine the following coded message: **15, 13, J, {(14, I), (1, 2)}, S** *[handwritten: building]*

Now examine the following sentences and try to determine the most likely interpretation of the code.

A   People repeated their conversations positively, as they were opposite to their office.

B   You can only come out of the house, if you speak nicely to me.

C   If you do not get out of the flat, I will never speak to you again.

D   She went back inside the house, as she was being called names.

E   The company's name was very offensive.

future conditional (building structure)

shade fire

Example 12 *(opposite le)*

Examine the following coded message: **12, 15, (S, G), (1, M), ⊠, E, T**

Now examine the following sentences and try to determine the most likely interpretation of the code.

A She was shocked when the house caught fire, all the rooms were black.

B He will be shocked if you ever painted his bedroom hot pink.

C The house is a shade of hot pink.

D She will be shocked if you ever painted her bedroom hot pink.

E She was surprised when she saw the bedrooms were a shade of shocking pink.

Example 13

Examine the following coded message: **11, P, T, A, (Q, X), J**

Now examine the following sentences and try to determine the most likely interpretation of the code.

A I will injure my leg if I don't run from the fire tomorrow.

B We will get injured if we come near the fire.

C Individuals should run from fires to avoid getting hurt.

D I was running, otherwise the fire would have burned me.

E I injured my ankle as I ran away from the fire.

past harm fire sprint

(body part) individual

Justifications of Decision Analysis Practice Answers

Example 1	**Answer A**

C, L, U, (10, T)

The code combines the words: apparatus, oxygen, senses, increased and fire.

Option A **Is the correct answer; it makes use of all of the coded words. 'Apparatus' is replaced with 'bunsen burner', 'senses' is replaced with 'smelt', 'oxygen' is replaced with 'gas' and 'increased, fire' are replaced with 'very hot'.**

Option B Does not include definition of encoded word 'senses'. Also combines air with increase which is not in the code.

Option C Does not include a definition of the encoded word 'senses' and introduces the word 'pipes'.

Option D Introduces the word 'you' and does not make use of the word 'increased'.

Option E Ignores the word 'increased' and 'fire'.

Example 2	**Answer C**

(1, W), N, F, (1, M), 13

The code combines the words: (opposite, take), human, crash, (opposite, he) and present.

Option A Introduces the word 'out' and ignores the words 'opposite, take'.

Option B Ignores the meaning of the words in brackets 'opposite, he', 'opposite, take' and introduces the word 'pulled'.

Option C **Although it introduces 'only' it is the best match because it makes use of all the codes. The 'opposite, take' is replaced with 'give', the 'opposite, he' is replaced with 'she', 'crash' is replaced with 'break' and 'past' is used to define the sentence being set in the past tense.**

Option D   Ignores the words in brackets 'opposite, take' and introduces the words 'out' and 'only'.

Option E   Uses all of the coded words, but also introduces the words 'kiss of life'.

Example 3   **Answer E**

E, (1, B), T, 11

The code combines the words: shade, (opposite, night), fire and past.

Option A   Ignores the rule of the words in brackets 'opposite, night'.

Option B   Uses all of the coded words, but introduces the word 'happened'.

Option C   Uses the coded words but introduces the word 'no'.

Option D   Introduces the words 'no' and 'protection'. This option also ignores the words in brackets 'opposite, night'.

Option E   **Is the correct answer. The word 'shade' is replaced with the colour 'red', 'opposite, night' is replaced with 'day', 'fire' is replaced with 'hot' and the sentence is set in the 'past' tense.**

Example 4   **Answer B**

10, K, L, B, (1, B), 12

The code combines the words: increased, liquid, oxygen, night, (opposite, night) and future

Option A   The sentence is set in the past tense instead of the future tense and ignores 'oxygen'.

Option B   **Is the correct answer. It uses all of the codes and rules within the brackets and is set in the 'future' tense. The word 'rain' is a metaphor for 'liquid', 'increased' is replaced by 'a lot' and 'oxygen' is replaced with 'air'.**

Option C	Uses the past tense and ignores the words 'oxygen' and 'opposite, night'.
Option D	Uses all of the encoded words however this option is set in the past tense and does not flow logically.
Option E	Uses the past tense and ignores the word 'night'.

Example 5   **Answers C and D**

15, 12, (K, 10), G, F

The code combines the words: conditional, future, (liquid, increased), structure and crash.

Option A	Uses the present tense and ignores the word 'crash'.
Option B	Uses the term 'liquid' three times within the sentence; 'rain', 'flooded', and 'water' and ignores the word 'crash'.
Options C & D	**Are the correct answers. Both options describe situations based on 'conditional' circumstances which may happen in the 'future'. In this instance the condition is that if it rains the bridge is more likely to fall. 'Liquid' is replaced by 'rain', the word 'heavily' is used to describe the rain fall 'increasing'. The word 'structure' is replaced by 'bridge' and finally 'crash' is replaced by the word 'fall'.**
Option E	Ignores the word 'crash' and is set in the present tense.

Example 6   **Answer B**

(14, H), 6, M, (14, I), 10, O, 13

The code combines the words: (plural, number), challenging, he, (plural, word), increased, achievement and present.

Option A	Ignores the encoded word 'increased' and is set in the past tense.

Option B	**Is the correct answer. The word 'maths' is used as a synonym for 'plural, number' and the word 'English' is used as a synonym for 'plural, word'. 'Difficult' is used as another definition of 'challenging' and 'increased' is replaced by 'very' to provide more emphasis on the definition of 'difficulty' on the examination – which is an 'achievement'.**
Option C	Uses all of the words and the tense is accurate, however the definition of the word 'number' is not in a 'plural' form.
Option D	The definition of 'number' is not in a 'plural' form and the sentence is set in the past tense.
Option E	Ignores the word 'he', the definition of 'number' is not in a 'plural' form and the sentence is set in the past tense.

Example 7	**Answers A and D**
	(14, M), U, 11, F, V, (1, B)
	The code combines the words: (plural, he), senses, past, crash, disaster and (opposite, night).
Option A	**Is the correct answer. The 'plural, he', is replaced with 'men', 'catastrophe' replaces 'disaster', the 'opposite, night' is replaced with 'day' and the word 'senses' is an individuals' four senses of sight, touch, hearing and smell. Within this scenario the sense is *sight*.**
Option B	The word 'he' is used and is therefore not plural. Also the word 'condition' has been introduced.
Option C	Ignores the definition of the words in brackets 'opposite, night'.
Option D	Uses all of the words and the tense is accurate, however the word 'more' has been introduced.
Option E	Introduces the word 'absolute', and ignores the word 'senses'.

Example 8	Answer C

10, 11, (1, M), O, W, ✄

The code combines the words: increased, past, (opposite, he), achievement, take and happy.

Option A	Ignores the word 'take' and is set in the present tense.
Option B	Ignores the rule of 'opposite, he'.
Option C	**Is the correct answer. It is set in the 'past' tense, 'happy' is replaced with 'content', 'take' is another interpretation of 'receive' and 'exam results' is a replacement for the word 'achievement'.**
Option D	Ignores the word 'take' and is set in the present tense.
Option E	Uses the word 'unhappy' instead of 'happy'.

Example 9	Answer E

(X, Q), (1, M), U, (T, V, K), 13, R

The code combines the words: (part, body), (opposite, he), senses, (fire, disaster, liquid), present and tremor.

Option A	Makes 'she' plural and describes a group of 'women' rather than an individual female. The word 'part' is also ignored.
Option B	Ignores any reference to the words 'fire' and 'part'. The scenario is also set in the past tense instead of the present tense.
Option C	Ignores the word 'part'.
Option D	Introduces the word 'fear'.
Option E	**Is the correct answer. 'body, part' is replaced with 'hands', 'shaking' replaces 'tremor' and the senses used within this scenario are the character's 'eyes' as she 'sees' the volcano erupt. Fire, disaster and liquid are combined within brackets to describe a 'volcano'. The scenario is in the present tense.**

Example 10   **Answer D**

O, (1, 2), (◉, E), (1, M)

The code combines the words: achievement, (opposite, positive), (sad, shade) and (opposite, he).

Option A   Ignores the rule of 'opposite, he'.

Option B   The words 'sad' and 'shade' are not combined together.

Option C   Mentions the word 'shade' twice, once with the word shade, and once with a separate word blue.

Option D   Is the correct answer, the words 'sad' and 'shade' are combined together which gives one word 'blue', which describes a 'sad' / 'negative' feeling. 'Achievement' is replaced with 'passing the course'.

Option E   The words 'sad' and 'shade' are not combined together.

Example 11   **Answer C**

15, 13, J, {(14, I), (1, 2)}, S

The code combines the words: conditional, present, individual, {(plural, word), (opposite, positive)} and building.

Option A   Introduces the word 'repeated', ignores the word 'individual' and uses the word 'people' instead. Also ignores the words in brackets – 'opposite, positive', and ignores conditional and not present tense.

Option B   Ignores the negative use of words, (opposite, positive).

Option C   Although it introduces 'get out' is the best match. The option is based on the 'condition' that if the other person does not come out of the flat (building), then he/she will stop (opposite, positive) talking (plural, word) to them. The sentence is set in the 'present' tense.

Option D   Is incorrect as the sentence is set in the past tense and is not based on a 'conditional' scenario.

Option E   Is set in the past tense and is not based on a 'conditional' scenario.

Example 12 – Answer D

12, 15, (S, G), (1, M), ⌧, E, T

The code combines the words: future, conditional, (building, structure), (opposite, he), surprised, shade and fire.

Option A   Set in the past tense and is not based on a 'conditional' scenario.

Option B   Uses all of the words, but ignores the rule of the 'opposite, he'. Also the word 'painted' is introduced.

Option C   Ignores many words; 'opposite to he', 'surprised', 'structure' and the scenario is not based on a 'conditional' future tense.

Option D   Although it introduces 'painted' is the best match. The scenario is based on the 'condition' that if you painted his/her bedroom hot pink they will be surprised. Therefore it is set in the future tense. The words 'building, structure' are combined to give the word 'bedroom', (which is a part of a house (building). 'Shaded' is replaced with 'pink' and 'fire' is replaced with 'hot' to give the emphasis of the colour.

Option E   Does not make reference to the word 'fire' and is set in the past tense.

Example 13 – Answer E

11, P, T A, (Q, X), J

The code combines the words: past, harm, fire, sprint, (body, part) and individual.

Option A   Is set in the future tense instead of the 'past' tense. Also the word 'tomorrow' is introduced.

Option B   'We' is used instead of an individual person. Ignores the following encoded words 'body, part' and 'sprinted'. Set in the future tense.

Option C   Ignores the words 'body, part', makes the word 'individual' plural and introduces the word 'avoid'. Also ignores past tense.

Option D   Ignores the word 'part'.

Option E   **Is the correct answer, as it is set in the past tense. The following encoded words are replaced: 'individual' is replaced with 'I', 'harm' is substituted for 'injured', 'sprint' is substituted for 'ran', 'body, part' are combined to give 'ankle' and 'fire' is kept in its original format.**

Chapter 7

The Non-Cognitive Analysis Subtest

The Non-Cognitive Analysis subtest identifies whether or not a candidate's personal profile matches their chosen career path. In general, the Non-Cognitive subtest is fairly similar to a personality test. The main purpose of this test is to establish whether or not a candidate will be happy and content within their career; whether they will be able to cope and manage with the daily pressures and constraints from being a student to a newly qualified medical or dental professional.

The Non-Cognitive Analysis subtest aims to explore aspects of a person's character that are thought to remain stable throughout their lifetime. The individual's pattern of behaviour, thoughts, feelings and emotions are all important concepts. The Non-Cognitive Analysis subtest aims to explore the following aspects:

- Robustness
- Empathy
- Integrity
- Honesty

Format of the Non-Cognitive Analysis subtest

The four concepts above will be identified by a questionnaire format in the UKCAT. Some questions will depict scenarios where candidates will be asked to decide what to do according to their morals, values and opinions. It is important to note that there are **no preferred answers**, and hence no answer is right or wrong. Candidates will be asked to choose an answer based on a scoring system. The choices will be presented as a series of options and candidates will need to choose an option which they believe closely fits their values and beliefs.

Other questions will include statements or pairs of statements of various concepts. These questions are specifically designed to measure a candidate's behaviour, attitudes, experiences and reactions to feelings of stress and well-being. With each question or statement candidates will be asked to specify how strongly they agree or disagree.

It is important that you answer the questions as truthfully as possible, as this test is designed to identify the 'real you'. In addition to this, it is vital that you do not answer the questions according to 'How you think you may want to be seen'. These specific types of test have a built-in mechanism which identifies inconsistencies in a candidate's answers. For example, some of the questions are purposely designed to assess the degree of honesty the questionnaire has been approached with. It is also essential that you acknowledge that not all candidates will receive the same questions, as these will be randomly selected from a larger set of possible questions.

The actual Non-Cognitive Analysis subtest will take you no longer than 30 minutes to complete. However it has not been stated by the UKCAT how many questions there are in total. Generally speaking the majority of personality questionnaires usually consist of approximately 100 to 150 items, in the given time limit. That said, it is only an estimate and hence you may find the number of items is actually less than the indicated estimate.

Illustrated below are examples of the types of questions you may find in the Non-Cognitive Analysis subtest. You may find it beneficial to work through these, in order to familiarise yourself with the content of this section of the UKCAT.

Summary of Non-Cognitive structure

This section of the UKCAT does not contain any 'Stem' specific questions. Instead there are various scenarios and statements which candidates are required to show their degree of agreement with.

Time limit = 30 minutes. There is no specific number of questions for this subtest.

Example 1

Tom, Lee and Joe are working together on a science experiment. Tom is tasked with recording the results while Lee and Joe carry out the experiment. After working on the experiment for a few hours, Lee notices that the information that Tom has written is incorrect. Lee tells Joe and they both realise they would have to start the whole experiment again. Lee suggests that they should tell Tom and get him out of their group. However Joe suggests that would be an unfair decision. Instead Joe suggests that they should tell Tom that it is someone else's turn to do the recording of the results. Lee feels that they would be lying, but Joe replies that they would not be hurting anyone else's feelings.

What is your opinion? How do you feel about each of the following statements?

There is no harm in lying if we are protecting the feelings of others.

Strongly Agree

Agree

Disagree

Strongly Disagree

Lying is always wrong.

Strongly Agree

Agree

Disagree

Strongly Disagree

It is always important to achieve the best marks, whatever it takes.

Strongly Agree

 Agree

Disagree

Strongly Disagree

The truth must be told, regardless of who gets hurt.

Strongly Agree

Agree

 Disagree

Strongly Disagree

Some achievements in life are more important than friendships.

Strongly Agree

Agree

Disagree

Strongly Disagree

A good friend will always tell the truth, be it good or bad.

Strongly Agree

Agree

Disagree

Strongly Disagree

Example 2

The following example contains statements about how you may behave in various situations and statements about how others behave. Read each of the statements carefully and quickly decide whether you think each statement is:

Definitely True

True on the whole

False on the whole

Definitely False

I know I am able to stick to deadlines under pressure.

Definitely True

~~True on the whole~~

False on the whole

Definitely False

My peers would describe me as a friendly and easygoing person.

Definitely True

~~True on the whole~~

False on the whole

Definitely False

I strive hard to overcome challenges and achieve

~~Definitely True~~

True on the whole

False on the whole

Definitely False

I have the ability to stick to deadlines whilst being under immense pressure.

Definitely True

~~True on the whole~~ (circled)

False on the whole

Definitely False

I would rather follow the opinions of the majority of the group rather than put forward my differing perspectives.

Definitely True

True on the whole

~~False on the whole~~ (circled)

Definitely False

Example 3

Another part of the subtest will include a section of paired statements which will represent opposing perspectives. Read the following statements and state your degree of agreement by ticking the box that satisfies your answer.

1.

I worry a lot about stressful work loads

I do not worry a lot about stressful workloads

2.

I start quarrels with others easily

I do not start quarrels with others easily

3.

I persevere until the task is finished

I do not persevere until the task is finished

4.

I adapt my behaviour to meet others' expectations

I never adapt my behaviour to meet others' expectations

5.

I trust people easily

I do not trust people easily

Chapter 8

Entire Mock UKCAT Exam

We would recommend that you complete the mock test under timed conditions and that you do not look at the answers until you have completed the test. The mock test should be completed in 90 minutes.

You will need to print the answer sheet which is available to download for free from www.Apply2Medicine.co.uk

PLEASE NOTE THERE IS NO NON-COGNITIVE SECTION IN THE MOCK TEST

Verbal Reasoning – 22 minutes

Question 1

> *Children are often not kind to each other; this can also be said for adults. This is simply the way the world revolves. Children need to learn and spend time together without adults interfering, in order to learn and develop a sense of consequence for their own actions. In recent times educational psychologists have proposed that the level of playground bullying has been over-exaggerated and parents should allow their children to learn and cope with name-calling and teasing in order for them to develop coping mechanisms to deal with crisis situations. Some childhood experts have argued that society is 'wrapping children up in cotton wool'. Parents, teachers, police, the government and wider society may all be to blame for over-exaggerating risk crises such as 'stranger danger' and 'drug abuse'.*
>
> *However, on the other side of this argument, an adult may perceive name calling as a petty matter although it may leave a child with detrimental consequences. To a certain degree the word 'bullying' may be excessively used and often adults may fail to differentiate this from what may be 'normal' falling out but is being perceived as bullying.*

A   Parents need to allow children to be more resilient.

B   The author feels playground bullying is overly exaggerated.

C   The idea that bullying is exaggerated is a controversial topic.

D   Psychologists believe that playground bullying is excessively over-stated.

Question 2

> Early results of a 12 million pound four-year study suggest that there are more benefits of eating organic food as opposed to non-organic food. Food items such as fruits, vegetables and milk seem to have much more nutrition than non-organic produce. Often these organic products have been shown to have higher levels of cancer-fighting properties and heart beneficial antioxidants.
>
> The results of the study suggest that organic food has up to 40% more antioxidants than non-organic products. Greater amounts were also found in organic milk, which was almost 20% higher than in organic food.
>
> These findings tend to contradict claims made by the UK Government's Food Standards Agency, which state that organic produce is equally as healthy as non-organic produce.

A   Organic milk has 60% more antioxidants than organic food.

B   Organic food is healthier than non-organic food.

C   The findings suggest that organic food is more beneficial than non-organic food.

D   An organic strawberry may have more antioxidants than a non-organic strawberry.

Question 3

> The world's largest search engine 'Google' is to ban adverts from companies which offer essay writing services. The internet company has informed companies regarding the ban which was due to be enforced in June 2007. This ban has been encouraged by a number of universities as these universities are very eager to identify 'cheaters'. This form of plagiarism almost certainly devalues the efforts of those students who work hard to achieve their qualifications.
>
> On the other side of this ban, essay writing companies believe that the ban will affect their legal business. Some companies have suggested that their services are simply a guide for individuals to follow; they do not expect students to hand in their essays as marked work. Virtually 90% of UK universities are believed to have plagiarism software in order to catch dishonest students.
>
> Essay writing companies join an increasing list of companies who promote content which is perceived to be inappropriate by Google, such as fake documents and adverts for tobacco.

A UK universities have plagiarism software which helps to identify cheaters.

B The enforced ban will decrease plagiarism.

C Essay writing companies may lose profits from the effects of the ban.

D UK universities encourage the ban.

Question 4

In computing a process is an illustration of a computer program that is being sequentially carried out. A single program is merely a submissive gathering of instructions; a process actually actions these instructions. Contemporary computer systems permit numerous processes to be gathered into memory at the same time through time-sharing and give a facade that they are being actioned at the same time even if there is just one processor. If there are multiple processors it may be possible to comprise a number of processes to be actioned simultaneously without the necessity for processor time-sharing.

Multiple processes may be related with the same program – each would execute and function with its own resources. A process coherent with a single instance of a program may advance and separate into multiple threads that may actually execute simultaneously through multi-tasking or multi-processing.

A A computer program is able to execute instructions.

B Contemporary computer systems allow numerous processes to be executed at the same time.

C Multiple processes are related to the same program.

D Multiple processors can have a number of processes being executed at the same time.

Question 5

Gross Domestic Product (GDP) is a crucial part of the UK National Accounts. It provides a calculation of the total economic activity in a region. In the third quarter of 2007, GDP increased by 0.8%, the same rate of growth as in the previous quarter.

Total production: Manufacturing increased by 0.2% in the third quarter in contrast to the second quarter where there was a rise of 0.8%. Electricity, gas and water showed growth of 1.0% in the third quarter compared with a 0.4% fall in the second quarter. Total services increased by 1.0% in the third quarter of 2007 in contrast to the previous quarter where there was a rise of 0.9%.

A   For six months the GDP remained consistent.

B   The rate of growth from April to June was the same as the rate of growth from July to September 2007.

C   The total production rate in the third quarter was higher than that in the second quarter.

D   The third quarter made more profit than the second quarter.

Question 6

It has been a controversial debate that half of the jobs which Labour introduced in 1997 have been filled by foreign workers. The Department of
Work and Pensions has claimed that over 52% of jobs have gone to foreign
workers. One most recent eye-opener has been that the government has
declared that more than 1.1 million overseas workers have come to Britain
in the past 10 years and not 8 million as previously disclosed.

National statistics provided by the Home Office have claimed that there
have been 1.5 million overseas workers over the last decade. However in
reply to this, the Department of Work and Pensions has claimed that the
extra 400,000 workers were British residents who were born overseas. With
such statistics, the findings seem to make a mockery of what the government had initially proposed – 'British jobs for every British worker'.

A   British workers have taken 48% of jobs.

B   Due to the controversial debate the government did not fully disclose
the statistics of foreigners.

C   The findings make a mockery of the Government's proposal of 'British
jobs for every British worker'.

D   The Home Office statistics are not a true representation of the total
number of overseas workers.

**YOU ARE NOW OVER THE HALFWAY STAGE OF THIS SECTION.
IDEALLY YOU SHOULD HAVE APPROXIMATELY 10 MINUTES LEFT**

(Please note this prompt will not be given in your actual test)

Question 7

> As she walked through the dark woods, she could feel the whisper of the wind blow across her face. The radiance of the sun peeked through the branches of the trees. The oak tree stood strong, facing the lake of swans. Towards the west stood an aged cottage house, amongst the perimeter of the building a pathway could be seen which led deeper into the darkness. Vanessa felt at peace, with the company of Mother Nature surrounding her. She walked towards the house and noted that towards her east stood a soaring fir tree. As she reached the doorstep of the house, she could see at the rear of the house the surface of Mount Sisilia. The ranges were intertwined but the two peaks could be briefly seen, which emphasised their individuality.

A The fir tree is on the left-hand side of the house.

B Mount Sisilia consists of two mountain ranges.

C Opposite the lake is an oak tree.

D The character in the passage is not afraid of the woods.

Question 8

> *The type and level of dyslexia varies from person to person. Approximately 60% of people with dyslexia suffer from phonological difficulties, and therefore have difficulty organising words from sounds, and the way they are written. This has often resulted in problems with reading, writing and spelling. One common feature is that people who have dyslexia often spell out words the way they sound, therefore making grammatical errors such as missing out silent letters and not following spelling rules.*
>
> *Dyslexia is usually noted in childhood, where children may confuse directional words and actions such as up and down, left or right, and in or out. During childhood they may also have difficulty with sequencing such as learning and memorising rhymes and number sequences.*
>
> *Dyslexia also continues throughout adulthood, and still affects sequencing and directional problems such as reading maps, difficulty with writing and reading tasks and dialling numbers on a telephone. Therefore, due to these difficulties with reading and spelling, individuals may find dictionaries and spell checkers difficult to understand.*

T

A   People with dyslexia may spell the word 'ghost' as 'gost', and miss out the letter 'H'.

C-T   B   Dyslexic children may have difficulty putting their shoes on correctly.

f   C   Maps cannot help individuals who suffer from dyslexia.

T   D   An individual who has dyslexia may find it difficult to write an essay.

Question 9

> *Younger people were more likely to take days off due to sickness than older*
> *employees. This was the case for both gender groups. Amongst 16–25 year*
> *old men 2.6% were more likely to take days off due to sickness. Of women*
> *from the same age category; 3.5% were more likely to take days off due to*
> *sickness.*
>
> *Women with no dependant children had the same sickness absence as*
> *women who had dependant children. Women whose children were aged*
> *between 5–10 years were more likely to take sickness absence than men*
> *(3.6%).*
>
> *The employees most likely to be sick worked in professional and technical*
> *occupations at an absence rate of 3.2%. This was followed by a rate of 2.8%*
> *in the elementary occupations, such as hospital porters, window cleaners*
> *and traffic wardens. In comparison the rate for women was 4.2%.*

C·T   A   Women are more likely to take days off due to sickness than men.

T   B   Employees of educational age are more likely to have sickness absences than older employees.

C·T   C   Professionals in stressful jobs, such as lawyers, are more likely to take days off.

T   D   Young people take more sickness absence than older people.

Question 10

> To be an effective leader, you need to have a vision and to know how you are going to bring people together to understand it. Charisma plays a vital role in leadership; charismatic leaders are admired by others and are concerned with others around them. A good leader also needs to understand when and when not to take risks, and how to portray success. Good leaders will usually pass down the glory to their teams, so that the teams feel satisfied with their winnings. When unforeseen circumstances come about, good leaders will also need to have the ability to claim a level of responsibility over strategies and related items which do not flow according to plan. True leaders are eager to offer power to get things done rather than hoarding power.

A   Good leaders should create a collective sense of achievement.

B   Good leaders should hand over complete power.

C   Charismatic leaders make better leaders.

D   Good leaders will need to claim responsibility over events that do not go according to plan.

Question 11

> The Smoke-free law aims to improve health in many ways as it reduces the risk of individuals suffering from the effects of passive smoking. There are over 4,000 chemicals in second-hand smoke. These are in forms of particles and gases, which often have poisonous properties that are known to cause cancer and heart problems. Within 30 minutes of exposure to second-hand smoke, blood flow to the heart is restricted. The Smoke-free law aims to reduce such harmful effects of second-hand smoke.
>
> The 'Smoke free law', passed by Parliament in 2006, makes virtually all enclosed public places and workplaces smoke-free. The law recognises individual rights to be protected from the harmful effects of smoke, and also aims to encourage smokers to quit. It has been suggested that reducing the exposure of cigarette smoke not only improves one's health, but also improves life expectancy.
>
> There are limited exemptions from the Smoke-free law. These regulations include bedrooms, hotels, care homes, prisons and various other 'live-in' premises. In the majority of cases, exemptions do not apply to the whole premises, but to certain 'designated rooms'.

A   The Smoke-free law will make people live longer.

B   Night staff working in a residential home are allowed to smoke in their own bedrooms.

C   There are 4,000 chemicals in second-hand smoke.

D   Public places and work places will abide by the Smoke-free law.

Quantitative Reasoning – 22 minutes

Carefully examine the codes below

A = 5.2	B = 3.6	C = 7	D = 8	E = 0.01

1   Solve the following equation: $D^3 \times C^2 = x^2$ and find the value of x. (Give your answer to one decimal place.)

   A   158.4

   B   158.3

   C   25,088

   D   2.50

   E   158.0

2   Solve the following equation: $(A^3 - 3) \times 2.2 = x$ and find the value of x^2. (Calculate your answer to one decimal place.)

   A   302.73

   B   302.7

   C   91,650.0

   D   91,650.05

   E   91,650.1

3   Solve the following equation: $(B \times C^2) \div 3 = x^2$ and find the value of x. (Calculate your answer to two decimal places.)

   A   7.668

   B   7.68

   C   7.667

   D   7.66

   E   7.67

4 **Solve the following equation: $(D^2 - 6) + (14 \times B) = x$ and find the value of x^3 (to one decimal place).**

A 108.4

B 1,273,760.7

C 1,373,760.7

D 1,723,760.0

E 1,273,706.7

A cake recipe serves eight people and includes the following ingredients.

Ingredients	Amount (grams)
Flour	750
Sugar	212.4
Butter	232.4
4 eggs	

5 **How much flour (in grams) would you need to bake a cake for 100 people?**

A 93.75

B 9,753

C 9,375

D 957

E 9,573

6   How much sugar will be required if the recipe was based for 7 people? (Give your answer in kilograms to three decimal places)

A   0.186

B   185.856

C   0.1858

D   0.1586

E   158.586

7   The recipe (for 8 people) is then modified to reduce the sugar content by 20%. How much sugar (in grams) will each person intake?

A   21.42

B   196.29

C   22.14

D   21.24

E   169.92

8   Using the same recipe, if 1,500 grams of flour is used, how many people will this cake recipe serve?

A   16.2

B   16

C   61

D   15

E   15.2

The table below shows a person's score on each game

Game	Score
1	20
2	30
3	60
4	10
5	20
6	60
7	60
8	70
9	20
10	10

9 What is the average score?

A 30

B 26

C 36

D 20

E 25

10 What is the median score?

A 50

B 25

C 55

D 20

E 35

11 **What is the range of the scores?**

    A   60

    B   50

    C   65

    D 55

    E   55.5

12 **If the mean score increases by 12.3%, what is the new mean score? (Calculate your answer to two decimal places.)**

    A   40.3

    B   40.34

    C   40.42

    D   40.43

    E   40.44

Carefully study the table below

Colour of door	Height of door (cm)					
	200–299	300–399	400–499	500–599	600–699	700–799
BLUE	56	24	42	100	912	100
GREEN	56	560	83	12	12	110
YELLOW	12	22	30	30	12	100

13 **How many green doors have a height of ≥ 600 cm?**

A   132

B   124

C   122

D   143

E   134

14 **How many blue doors are there with a height of ≤ 499 cm to yellow doors with a height of ≤ 399 cm? (Calculate your answer as a ratio.)**

A   17:61

B   61:30

C   61:17

D   71:16

E   16:71

15 **How many yellow doors are in there in total? (Give your answer as a percentage to two decimal places).**

A   9.6%

B   9.60%

C   09.06%

D   9.06%

E   06.09%

16 **What percentage of green doors have a height ≥ 600 cm? (Calculate your answer to two decimal places).**

A   14.65%

B   1.44%

C   1.47%

D   14.70%

E   1.43%

Carefully study the pie chart below

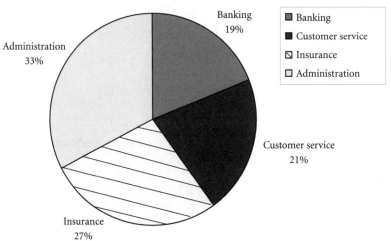

Pie chart showing number of staff employed in each sector
(Total number of staff 240)

17 **How many people are employed in the administration sector?**

A   79.2

B   97

C   97.008

D   79.008

E   79

18 **If staff numbers in the banking sector increase by 20%, what will the new total be in banking?**

A   54.7

B   55

C   55.8

D   44.5

E   44.4

19 If staff members in customer service increase by 35%, what will be the new percentage of staff employed in the customer service sector? (Calculate your answer to two decimal places.)

A   26.14%

B   26.15%

C   26.51%

D   26.41%

E   26.26%

20 How many more staff members are there in insurance than banking?

A   13

B   19

C   10

D   19.9

E   18.9

THIS IS THE HALFWAY STAGE OF THIS SECTION. IDEALLY YOU SHOULD HAVE APPROXIMATELY 11 MINUTES LEFT

(Please note this prompt will not be given in your actual test)

Carefully examine the codes below

A = −1	B = −3	C = 4.2	D = 5	E = 25.3	F = 3.9

21   Solve the following equation: $A + B^2 = x$ and find the value of x^2

    A   −100

    B   100

    C   −64

    D   8

    E   64

22   Solve the following equation: $(C + B) \div F = x$ and find the value of x (Calculate your answer to three decimal places.)

    A   0.308

    B   0.307

    C   1.846

    D   4.970

    E   3.431

23   Solve the following equation: $E^2 + B^3 = \sqrt{x}$ (Calculate your answer to one decimal place.)

    A   375,880

    B   357,878.4

    C   613.09

    D   375,879.3

    E   613.1

24 Solve the following equation: $(D + C^2) \div F = x^2$ and find the value of x (Calculate your answer to two decimal places.)

A   4.21

B   2.41

C   5.80

D   8.50

E   2.40

Carefully study the bar graph below.

Absence leave at Amber Cooperation in a period of three months

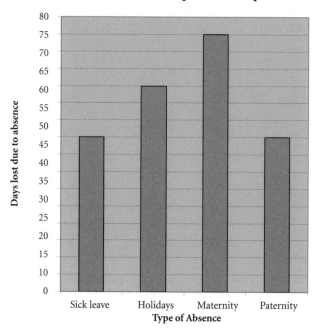

Loss per day of absence
Sick leave – £47.00
Holidays – £85.00
Maternity – £80.00
Paternity – £60.00

25 **How many more days have been lost due to people taking holidays as opposed to being off sick?**

A   51

B   60

C   50

D   15

E   61

26 **What is the ratio of days lost due to maternity leave to paternity leave?**

    A   9:15

    B   45:75

    C   75:45

    D   15:9

    E   5:3

27 **Month four sees an increase of 33.3% on average absence over the previous three months. How many more days were lost due to absence in month four?**

    A   15

    B   5

    C   14.9

    D   3.9

    E   26.1

28 **On average, how much did the company lose through paying all absence each month? (Give your answer in £.)**

    A   15,915

    B   5,360

    C   5,305

    D   3,752

    E   4,975

Examine the table below

Currency	Rate of exchange = Pound Sterling (£1)
American – Dollar	1.59 USD
Indian – Rupee	0.0856 R
French – Euro	1.45 €
Cuban – Peso	1.8 CUP
Bangladesh – Taka	0.6 BGL

29 How much is 150 USD American dollars worth in Pounds sterling (£)?

A £94.33

B £49.36

C £94.34

D £49.37

E £94.30

30 The exchange rate of American dollars changes to 1.805 dollars to the pound. How many more dollars do you get to the pound. (Calculate your answer as a percentage.)

A 10.5

B 15.3

C 88.1

D 11.9

E 13.5

31 What is the exchange rate if $120.89 was exchanged for £89.00? (Calculate your answer to two decimal places).

A   1.35

B   1.36

C   1.63

D   0.136

E   1.360

32 How many Bangladesh Takas can be bought with £100.61? (Calculate your answer to two decimal places.)

A   60.37

B   167.68

C   168.86

D   60.40

E   60.49

33 Reduce the following fraction into its simplest form 27/108

A   9/36

B   36/9

C   4/3

D   4/1

E   1/4

34 **Add the following fractions 3/8 + 1/5**

 A 46/80

 B 23/40

 C 4/8

 D 3/7

 D 31/360

35 **Convert 11/4 into a mixed fraction**

 A 2/3

 B 2¾

 C ¾2

 D 2⁴/₃

 E 4²/₃

36 **Convert 3²/₅ into an improper fraction.**

 A 17/5

 B 17/7

 C 5/17

 D 3/17

 E 17/3

37 **A vehicle travels 360 miles in four hours. What was the speed of the vehicle (in miles per hour)?**

 A 80

 B 72

 C 90

 D 92

 E 70

38 A vehicle travels 120 miles at 60 miles per hour, how long did the journey take? (Calculate your answer in minutes.)

A   120

B   130

C   125

D   135

E   140

39 A vehicle travels 150 miles at 50 miles per hour, then stops for 15 minutes, and then travels 160 miles at 40 miles per hour. What was the total duration of the whole journey? (Calculate your answer in minutes.)

A   425

B   325

C   435

D   335

E   420

40 A truck driver travels for 2 hours at an average speed of 70 miles an hour, he then hits road works and has to reduce his speed to 30 miles an hour, for 1.5 hours until he reaches his destination. How long was the driver's journey?

A   185 miles

B   140 miles

C   350 miles

D   150 miles

E   155 miles

Abstract Reasoning – 16 Minutes

Question 1

Set A

Set B

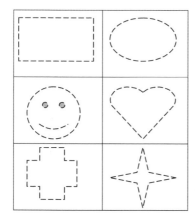 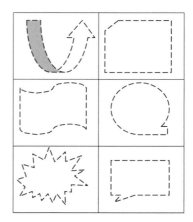

Test shape 1

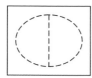

A ✓

Test shape 2

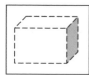

neither ✓

Test shape 3

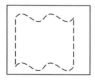

A X B

Test shape 4

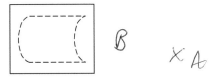

ℬ   × A

Test shape 5

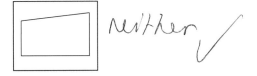

Neither ✓

Question 2

[handwritten] 1 heart 3 stars
3 stars 1 heart

Set A   **Set B**

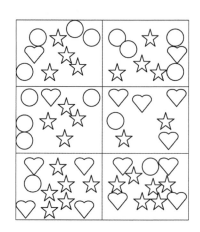

Test shape 1

  [handwritten] A ✓

Test shape 2

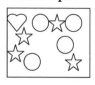 *[handwritten]* B ✓

Test shape 3

[handwritten] B ✓

Test shape 4

Neither ✓

Test shape 5

B ✓

Question 3

Set A   Set B

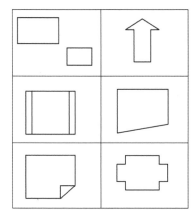   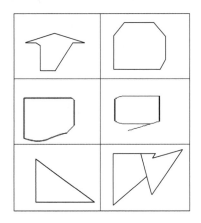

Test shape 1

 Neither

Test shape 2

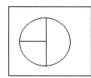 Neither

Test shape 3

 B

Test shape 4

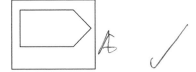

A ✓

Test shape 5

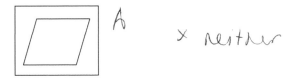

A

✗ neither

Question 4

Set A   Set B

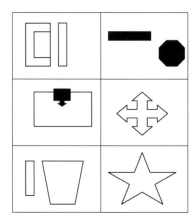

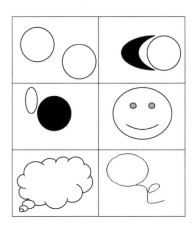

Test shape 1

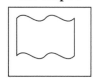

B ✗ Neither

Test shape 2

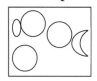

B ✓

Test shape 3

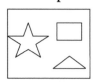

B ✗ A

Test shape 4

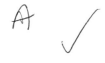

neither ✓

Test shape 5

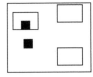

A ✓

Question 5

Set A	Set B

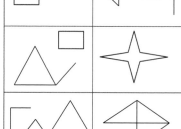

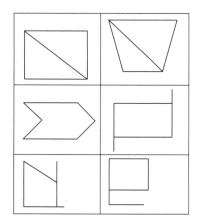

Test shape 1

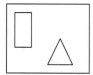

A ✗ Neither

Test shape 2

B ✓

Test shape 3

Neither ✗

Test shape 4

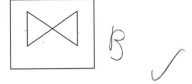

B ✓

Test shape 5

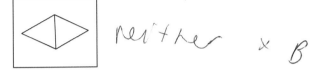

neither x B

Question 6

<table>
<tr><td align="center">**Set A**</td><td align="center">**Set B**</td></tr>
</table>

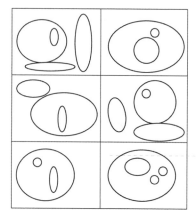 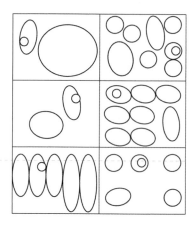

Test shape 1

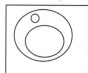

Test shape 2

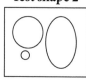

Test shape 3

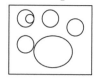

Test shape 4

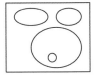

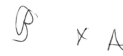

Test shape 5

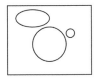

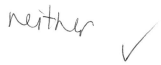

Question 7

<table>
<tr><td align="center">**Set A**</td><td align="center">**Set B**</td></tr>
</table>

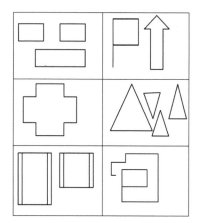 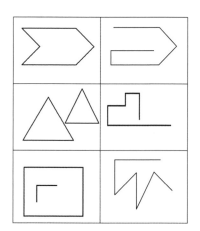

Test shape 1

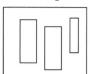

B × A

Test shape 2

A ✗ neither

Test shape 3

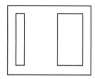

A ✓

Test shape 4

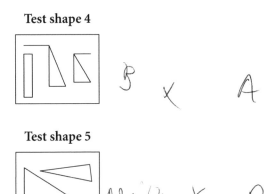

Test shape 5

**YOU ARE NOW OVER THE HALFWAY STAGE OF THIS SECTION.
IDEALLY YOU SHOULD HAVE APPROXIMATELY 7.5 MINUTES LEFT**

(Please note this prompt will not be given in your actual test)

Question 8

Set A

Set B

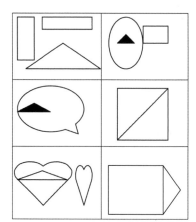
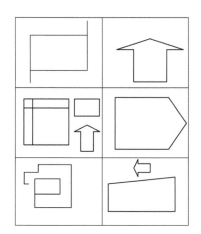

Test shape 1

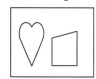

A ✗ neither

Test shape 2

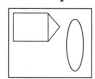

A ✓

Test shape 3

B ✗ A

Test shape 4

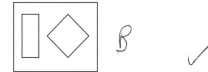

β ✓

Test shape 5

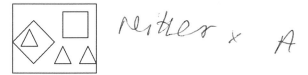

Neither x   A

Question 9

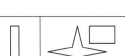

Set A   **Set B**

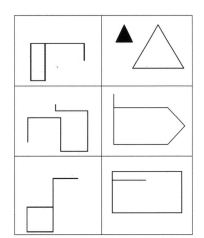

Test shape 1

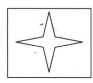

neither ✓

Test shape 2

B ✓

Test shape 3

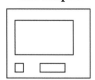

A ✓

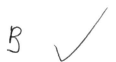

Test shape 4

Neither ✗ A

Test shape 5

Neither ✓

Question 10

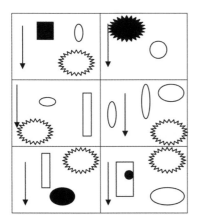

Set A

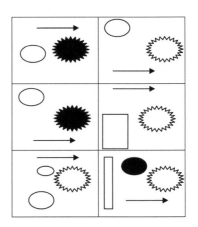

Set B

Test shape 1

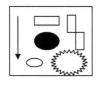

Test shape 2

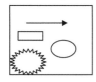

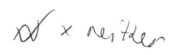

Test shape 3

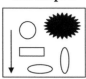

Test shape 4

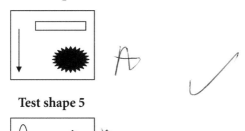

A ✓

Test shape 5

neither ✗   *B*

Question 11

Set A   **Set B**

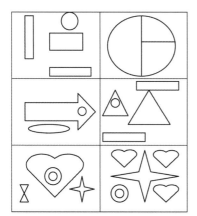 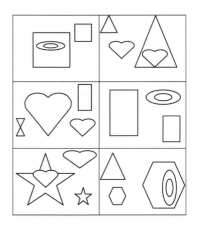

Test shape 1

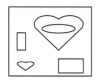

B ✓

Test shape 2

A ✗ *B*

Test shape 3

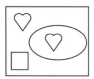

B ✗ neither

Test shape 4

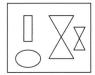
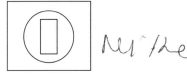

x A

Test shape 5

A

X B

Question 12

Set A	Set B

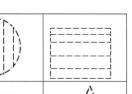

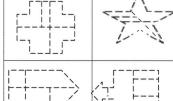

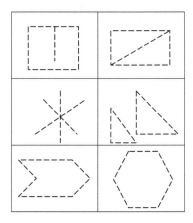

Test shape 1

A

Test shape 2

B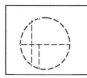

Test shape 3

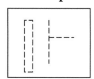

B

Test shape 4

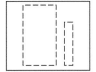

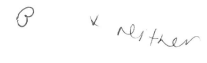

B × neither

Test shape 5

neither ✓

Question 13

Set A	Set B

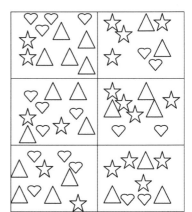

Test shape 1 4 star
2 tri

B

4 star
2 heart

Test shape 2

B

Test shape 3

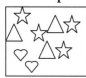

neither

Test shape 4

Test shape 5

46/65

Decision Analysis – 30 Minutes

Scenario

A group of archaeologists have discovered a hidden pyramid. They have found hieroglyphics on the walls which shows various codes. The team have managed to decode some of the messages; these are presented in the table below. Your task is to examine particular codes or sentences and then choose the best interpretation of the code from one of five possible choices.

You will find that, at times, the information you have is either incomplete or does not make sense. You will then need to make your best judgement based on the codes rather than what you expect to see or what you think is reasonable. There will always be a best answer which makes the most sense based on all the information presented. It is important that you understand that this test is based on judgements rather than simply applying rules and logic.

General Operating Codes	Basic codes	Verbs
1 = Antonym	A = Sea	♎ = Dining
2 = Present	B = Oxygen	= Drinking
3 = Past	C = Person	♑ = Brawling
4 = Future	D = Sun	= Seeing
5 = Increase	E = Night	♌ = Conversing
6 = Unite	F = Cold	☹ = Listening
7 = Plural	G = Today	♱ = Smiling
8 = Attribute	H = Tomorrow	☝ = Trusting
9 = Conditional	I = Weapon	✿ = Cope
10 = Open	J = Creature	
11 = Positive	K = Hazard	
12 = Weak	L = She	
13 = Frequently	M = Run	
	N = Emotion	
	O = Building	
	P = Drop	
	Q = Jungle	
	R = Escape	
	S = Triumph	
	T = Move	

ɔhe (attribute ɔea) drop past listening

Question 1

Examine the following coded message: **L, (8, A), P, 3, ⊗**

Now examine the following sentences and try to determine the most likely interpretation of the code.

A   She can hear the raindrops falling.

B   She listened to her past drop into the sea.

C   She dropped her past into the sea.

D   She listened to the rain falling.

E   She was listening to the music of the waves.

Ɍun (attribute oxygen) (attribute sea) past

Question 2

Examine the following coded message: **D, (8, B), (8, A), 3**

Now examine the following sentences and try to determine the most likely interpretation of the code.

A   The sun dried up the sea.

B   The sun dried up the rain.

C   There is no oxygen in the sea.

D   There is no air in the sea, but there is where the sun is.

E   There is more air near the sun than in water.

future (atonym cold)(atonym night.)
Question 3
tomorrow sun increase

Examine the following coded message: **4, (1, F), (1, E) H, D, 5**

Now examine the following sentences and try to determine the most likely interpretation of the code.

A   It will be a very hot, sunny day tomorrow.

B   It will be a hot and sunny day tomorrow.

C   It is a very sunny day tomorrow.

D   Tomorrow will be a very hot day.

E   It is going to be a very hot sunny day.

Question 4

Examine the following coded message: **L, M, O, 5 (A, 8), 2**

Now examine the following sentences and try to determine the most likely interpretation of the code.

A   She ran under the building as it was raining.

B   She is running to the house as it is raining heavily.

C   She ran towards her house which was near the sea.

D   She ran towards the building as the rain was falling heavily.

E   She will run under the buildings if the rain falls heavily.

She run building increase

(Sea attribute.)   present

future (Sea attribute) jungle (increase hazard)

Question 5 conditional (weather Create Player)

Examine the following coded message: **4, (A, 8), Q, (5, K) 9, (J, 7)**

Now examine the following sentences and try to determine the most likely interpretation of the code.

A   If it floods in the jungle will be very dangerous for the animals.

B   The rain increased in the jungle and became dangerous for the animals.

C   The mammals caused a large hazard in the sea.

D   The flood will be dangerous for the inhabitants living in the jungle.

E   The sea is a large hazard for the animals in the jungle.

Question 6

Examine the following coded message: **(A, 8), (7, C, O), 2**

Now examine the following sentences and try to determine the most likely interpretation of the code.

A   People were behind the building near the river.

B   The church is across the lake.

C   People were in the building as they saw the attributes of the sea.

D   The community centre was across the lake.

E   The lake was near the church.

Question 7

Examine the following coded message: **K, (7, C, O), (8, B) 3, R**

Now examine the following sentences and try to determine the most likely interpretation of the code.

A   People were trying to escape from the building.

B   People were trying to escape from the dangerous gas.

C   The office is dangerous as there is a gas leak.

D   People avoided the office due to the gas leak.

E   The office was dangerous as there was a gas leak.

Question 8

Examine the following coded message: **Ϡ, 9, (7, C), 3, (1, E), □**

Now examine the following sentences and try to determine the two most likely interpretations of the code.

A   The soldiers could have carried on with the battle had it been in the day.

B   They could have seen more if they had fought in the daylight.

C   The soldiers could have seen more if they had fought in the day.

D   The soldiers fought more in the day than in the night.

E   They could have seen more in the day than in the night.

Question 9

Examine the following coded message: ⊗, (J, 7), (1, 11, N), L, 3

Now examine the following sentences and try to determine the most likely interpretation of the code.

A   She felt frightened as she saw the animals come towards her.

B   She felt negative as she left the animals.

C   She was frightened as she heard the animals.

D   She felt a negative emotion as she heard the mammals.

E   She will be frightened once she hears the animals coming towards her.

Question 10

Examine the following coded message: S, (1, 5), 9 (1, ♪), (7, C), 2

Now examine the following sentences and try to determine the most likely interpretation of the code.

A   We will not succeed as we mistrust each other.

B   People will only succeed if they trust each other.

C   Mistrusting each other leads to a lack of success.

D   Success is less likely to come from mistrust.

E   If we are to doubt each other, then we are less likely to succeed.

Question 11

Examine the following coded message: **9, H, 5 (1, F), (7, C), A, 2, (5, ⊠)**

Now examine the following sentences and try to determine the most likely interpretation of the code.

A   People will drink a lot of water tomorrow if it is hot.

B   People drink a lot of water when it is hot.

C   People will go to the sea if it is hot tomorrow.

D   People will drink a lot of water if it is very hot today.

E   People will drink a lot of water if it is very hot.

Question 12

Examine the following coded message: **9, 4, S, (L, 1), ✝**

Now examine the following sentences and try to determine the most likely interpretation of the code.

A   He will be happy if he passes his exams.

B   He was very happy when he passed his exams.

C   He will be very happy with his future successes.

D   She will be very happy if she succeeds.

E   He will be smiling at his successes.

Question 13

Examine the following coded message: **(C, 7, O), (C, 7), 3**

Now examine the following sentences and try to determine the most likely interpretation of the code.

A   There will be a group of people at the church.

B   There was a crowd of people in the building.

C   There was a group of people in the buildings.

D   There is a group of people in the church.

E   There was a crowd of people at the community centre.

THIS IS THE HALFWAY STAGE OF THIS SECTION. IDEALLY YOU SHOULD HAVE APPROXIMATELY 15 MINUTES LEFT

(Please note this prompt will not be given in your actual test)

Question 14

Examine the following coded message: **(7, C), R, Q, (K, J, 7)**

Now examine the following sentences and try to determine the most likely interpretation of the code.

A   I made a quick getaway from the dangerous mammals in the jungle.

B   The group made a getaway from the mammals in the rainforest.

C   The tribe made a getaway from the dangerous animals in the rainforest.

D   The group escaped from the animals in the jungle.

E   The group made a quick getaway from the dangerous animals in the jungle.

Question 15

Examine the following coded message: **D, C (8, A), (N, 11) 5, (1, 11, N)**

Now examine the following sentences and try to determine the most likely interpretation of the code.

A   People feel very happy when it is sunny but sad when they are near the sea.

B   I only feel very positive when it is sunny near the sea.

C   I only feel sad when it rains but I am happy when it is sunny.

D   I feel very happy when I am near the sun and sad when it goes.

E   I only feel very happy when it is sunny and sad when it rains.

Question 16

Examine the following coded message: **(1, 11) N, C, (A, ♎), ♎**

Now examine the following sentences and try to determine two of the most likely interpretations of the code.

A   I like the flavour of fish.

B   I dislike the taste of fish.

C   I dislike the taste of seafood.

D   I feel like eating near the sea.

E   I loathe eating out in the rain.

Question 17

Examine the following coded message: (C, 7), (I ,7) 3, Ⴗ

Now examine the following sentences and try to determine the most likely interpretation of the code.

A   I prepared for battle.

B   I prepared for battle with my missiles.

C   The soldiers will use their guns as they fight.

D   The police force will prepare for battle.

E   The military used their arms as they prepared for conflict.

Question 18

Examine the following coded message: 2, (7, C), ♂, ♌

Now examine the following sentences and try to determine the most likely interpretation of the code.

A   Talkative people are never trusted.

B   Conversations lead to trust.

C   Trust first comes from verbal communication.

D   To maintain trust amongst staff it is important to communicate verbally.

E   People who are trusting tend to talk and listen.

Question 19

Examine the following coded message: **5 (8, A), (7, C, O), K, 4**

Now examine the following sentences and try to determine the most likely interpretation of the code.

A   The heavy rain was dangerous for people.

B   The flood will make the library dangerous.

C   The sea was hazardous for peoples' homes.

D   The flood will be dangerous for people.

E   The sea will be nearby and this will make the church dangerous.

Question 20

Examine the following coded message: **C (1, 11) ⊠, 13, (7, C, ⊠) 5**

Now examine the following sentences and try to determine the most likely interpretation of the code.

A   I like to drink regularly with my friends.

B   I do not drink regularly.

C   I am more of a social drinker than a regular drinker.

D   I regularly enjoy drinking and socialising with others.

E   I do not enjoy regularly drinking or socialising with others.

Question 21

Examine the following sentence: 'I will be happy to speak to you only if you listen to what I have to say'.

Now examine the following codes and try to determine the most likely interpretation of the sentence.

A C, 9, ✟, 4, ☹, ♌

B C, ✟, 2, ☹, ♌

C 9, C 2, ☹, ♌

D J, C, 9, ✟, 2, ☹, ♌

E C, C, 9, 9, ✟, 2, 2, ☹, ♌

Question 22

Examine the following sentence: 'People are dropping like flies from the heat'.

Now examine the following codes and try to determine the most likely interpretation of the sentence.

A (7, C) (7, J), 2, (1, F)

B (7, C) (7, J), 2

C (7, C) 7, J, 2, (1, F)

D (7, C) (7, J) P, 2, (1, F)

E C, (7, J) P, 2, (1, F)

Question 23

Examine the following sentence: 'Grin and bear it'.

Now examine the following codes and try to determine the most likely interpretation of the sentence.

A ✝, ✿

B J, ✝, ✿

C ✿, ✿, ✝, ✿

D ✿, A

E (✿, ✝)

Question 24

Examine the following sentence: 'The tide is very strong today and is dangerous'.

Now examine the following codes and try to determine the most likely interpretation of the sentence.

A A, T, 1, (12, G, K), 2

B (A, T), (1, 12), G, K, 2

C (A, T), (1, 12), G, K, 4

D (A, T), 12, G, K, 2

E A, T, 1, 12, G, K, 2

Question 25

Examine the following sentence: 'She was fighting for breath as she ran home'.

Now examine the following codes and try to determine the most likely interpretation of the sentence.

A   3, M, L, ℅, O

B   L, 3, L, ℅, 3, B, M, O

C   L, ℅, 3, B, M, O

D   L, 3, B, M, O

E   L, ℅, 4, B, M, O

Question 26

Examine the following sentence: 'He was happy to see his gift'.

Now examine the following codes and try to determine the most likely interpretation of the sentence.

A   L, 3, ✞,   , 2

B   1, 3, L, ✞,

C   (1, L), 3,

D   F, (1, L), 3, ✞,

E   (1, L), 3, ✞,   , 2

Verbal Reasoning
Answers and Justifications

Question 1

> *Children are often not kind to each other; this can also be said for adults. This is simply the way the world revolves. Children need to learn and spend time together without adults interfering, in order to learn and develop a sense of consequence for their own actions. In recent times educational psychologists have proposed that the level of playground bullying has been over-exaggerated and parents should allow their children to learn and cope with name-calling and teasing in order for them to develop coping mechanisms to deal with crisis situations. Some childhood experts have argued that society is 'wrapping children up in cotton wool'. Parents, teachers, police, the government and wider society may all be to blame for over-exaggerating risk crises such as 'stranger danger' and 'drug abuse'.*
>
> *However, on the other side of this argument, an adult may perceive name calling as a petty matter although it may leave a child with detrimental consequences. To a certain degree the word 'bullying' may be excessively used and often adults may fail to differentiate this from what may be 'normal' falling out but is being perceived as bullying.*

A *Parents need to allow children to be more resilient.*

Answer: True

It is stated in the passage that parents should allow their children to learn with name calling and teasing in order to develop their coping mechanisms.

B *The author feels playground bullying is overly exaggerated.*

Answer: Can't tell

In the passage it is stated that playground bullying is overly exaggerated; however, the author's views and perceptions are not given.

C *The idea that bullying is exaggerated is a controversial topic.*

Answer: True

Although there is no direct reference to the word controversial, there are various inconclusive and opposing views. Based on this reason it is fair to say that the above statement is true.

D   Psychologists believe that playground bullying is excessively overstated.

Answer: False

We are not given information about the beliefs of psychologists in general as stated above by the statement; instead we are given information regarding specific types of psychologists, i.e. educational psychologists.

Question 2

> *Early results of a 12 million pound four-year study suggest that there are more benefits of eating organic food as opposed to non-organic food. Food items such as fruits, vegetables and milk seem to have much more nutrition than non-organic produce. Often these organic products have been shown to have higher levels of cancer-fighting properties and heart beneficial antioxidants.*
>
> *The results of the study suggest that organic food has up to 40% more antioxidants than non-organic products. Greater amounts were also found in organic milk, which was almost 20% higher than in organic food.*
>
> *These findings tend to contradict claims made by the UK Government's Food Standards Agency, which state that organic produce is equally as healthy as non-organic produce.*

A   Organic milk has 60% more antioxidants than organic food.

Answer: False

Organic milk has *up to* 20% more antioxidants than organic food (which have up to 40%); and therefore equates to *up to* 60% rather than exactly 60%.

B   Organic food is healthier than non-organic food.

Answer: False

In the passage it is *suggested* that organic food *may be* more nutritious than non-organic food through the use of the word 'seem'. The passage does not contain information which implies that organic food is unquestionably healthier.

C *The findings suggest that organic food is more beneficial than non-organic food.*

Answer: Can't tell

We are only given information about the early results of the study; the complete results of the study are not evident, and this therefore means that there is insufficient information to confirm the above statement.

D *An organic strawberry may have more antioxidants than a non-organic strawberry.*

Answer: True

Based on the information given in the passage it is possible that organic food such as fruit may have more antioxidants than non-organic food. From this assumption we are able to say the above statement is true, even though this particular example is not illustrated in the passage.

Question 3

> *The world's largest search engine 'Google' is to ban adverts from companies which offer essay writing services. The internet company has informed companies regarding the ban which was due to be enforced in June 2007. This ban has been encouraged by a number of universities as these universities are very eager to identify 'cheaters'. This form of plagiarism almost certainly devalues the efforts of those students who work hard to achieve their qualifications.*
>
> *On the other side of this ban, essay writing companies believe that the ban will affect their legal business. Some companies have suggested that their services are simply a guide for individuals to follow; they do not expect students to hand in their essays as marked work. Virtually 90% of UK universities are believed to have plagiarism software in order to catch dishonest students.*
>
> *Essay writing companies join an increasing list of companies who promote content which is perceived to be inappropriate by Google, such as fake documents and adverts for tobacco.*

A **UK universities have plagiarism software which helps to identify cheaters.**

Answer: False

The statement refers to all UK universities; however in the passage it is stated that *virtually 90%* of UK universities have such software. In other words there is a possibility that the remaining 10% may not have the plagiarism software.

B **The enforced ban will decrease plagiarism.**

Answer: Can't tell

We are given information on what the ban is trying to achieve, but we are not provided with information on the actual effects of the ban. Hence, we are unable to conclude the above statement.

C **Essay writing companies may lose profits from the effects of the ban.**

Answer: Can't tell

We are told that the ban may affect essay writing companies but we are not provided with information on *how* it will affect such companies. For this reason we are unable to infer any conclusions from the above statement.

D **UK universities encourage the ban.**

Answer: False

The above statement generalises that *all* universities encourage the ban rather than, as the passage states, '*a number of universities*' encourage the ban. Or in other words, a certain number of universities encourage the ban. For this reason the above statement is false.

Question 4

In computing a process is an illustration of a computer program that is being sequentially carried out. A single program is merely a submissive gathering of instructions; a process actually actions these instructions. Contemporary computer systems permit numerous processes to be gathered into memory at the same time through time-sharing and give a facade that they are being actioned at the same time even if there is just one processor. If there are multiple processors it may be possible to comprise a number of processes to be actioned simultaneously without the necessity for processor time-sharing.

Multiple processes may be related to the same program – each would execute and function with its own resources. A process coherent with a single instance of a program may advance and separate into multiple threads that may actually execute simultaneously through multi-tasking or multi-processing.

A   A computer program is able to execute instructions.

Answer: False

The above statement is incorrect as a computer program is simply a 'submissive gathering of instructions', and the 'process actually actions these instructions'. Therefore it is the process that executes these instructions.

B   Contemporary computer systems allow numerous processes to be executed at the same time.

Answer: False

The above statement contradicts what is being suggested in the passage. The statement proposes that numerous processes can be executed or actioned at the same time, when in actual fact it is stated in the passage that contemporary computer systems give a 'facade' or an illusion that the numerous processes are actioned simultaneously. For this reason the statement is false.

C   Multiple processes are related to the same program.

Answer: False

The above statement is false, as it is stated in the passage 'Multiple processes *may be* related with the same program'; in other words there is a chance that the processes and programs might be related, but this is not definite.

D   Multiple processors can have a number of processes being executed at the same time.

Answer: True

It is stated in the passage 'If there are multiple processors it may be possible to effect a number of processes to be actioned simultaneously'.

Question 5

> Gross Domestic Product (GDP) is a crucial part of the UK National Accounts. It provides a calculation of the total economic activity in a region. In the third quarter of 2007, GDP increased by 0.8%, the same rate of growth as in the previous quarter.
>
> Total production: Manufacturing increased by 0.2% in the third quarter in contrast to the second quarter where there was a rise of 0.8%. Electricity, gas and water showed growth of 1.0% in the third quarter compared with a 0.4% fall in the second quarter. Total services increased by 1.0% in the third quarter of 2007 in contrast to the previous quarter where there was a rise of 0.9%.

A   For six months the GDP remained consistent.

Answer: Can't tell

We are given information about the 'rate' of growth for GDP which remained consistent for the second and third quarter of 2007; however we are not given information on the definite 'total' of the GDP, and for this reason we are unable to conclude the above statement.

B   The rate of growth from April to June was the same as the rate of growth from July to September 2007.

Answer: True

As mentioned in the previous justification, we are given information about the rate of growth which increased by 0.8% in the second and third quarters of 2007. The second quarter of a year includes the months April, May and June, and the third quarter of a year includes the months July, August and September. Therefore the above statement is true.

C   *The total production rate in the third quarter was higher than that in the second quarter.*

Answer: True

Under the heading of 'Total Production' there are various production rates from the following divisions:

Division	Second quarter	Third quarter
Manufacturing	(+) Increase of 0.8%	(+) Increase of 0.2%
Electricity, Gas and Water	(-) Decrease of 0.4%	(+) Increase of 1.0%
Total services	(+) Increase of 0.9%	(+)Increase of 1.0%
Total increase of production	**1.3%**	**2.2%**

We need to first add the total production rates for each quarter. It is also important to subtract the percentage decrease of the production rate as depicted in the table where there is a 0.4% decrease in the second quarter for Electricity, Gas and Water. We are then able to see that there was a higher production rate in the third quarter than the second quarter.

D   *The third quarter made more profit than the second quarter.*

Answer: Can't tell

We are not given information detailing profits; therefore we are unable to conclude the above statement.

Question 6

> It has been a controversial debate that half of the jobs which Labour in-
> troduced in 1997 have been filled by foreign workers. The Department of
> Work and Pensions has claimed that over 52% of jobs have gone to foreign
> workers. One most recent eye-opener has been that the government has
> declared that more than 1.1 million overseas workers have come to Britain
> in the past 10 years and not 8 million as previously disclosed.
>
> National statistics provided by the Home Office have claimed that there
> have been 1.5 million overseas workers over the last decade. However in
> reply to this, the Department of Work and Pensions has claimed that the
> extra 400,000 workers were British residents who were born overseas. With
> such statistics, the findings seem to make a mockery of what the govern-
> ment had initially proposed – 'British jobs for every British worker'.

A   48% of jobs have gone to British workers.

Answer: False

In the passage it is stated that *over* 52% of jobs have gone to foreign workers.
Therefore the percentage given in the statement should be lower, as there
are *over 52%* .

**B   Due to the controversial debate the government did not fully disclose
the statistics of foreigners.**

Answer: Can't tell

At the beginning of the passage it is stated that the debate is of a controversial nature; in addition to this the government has declared differing numbers of overseas workers. However the reasons why the government did not
fully disclose the actual numbers are not given and hence we are unable to
conclude the above statement.

**C   The findings make a mockery of the Government's proposal of 'British
jobs for every British worker'.**

Answer: False

In the passage it is suggested that the findings give the impression of making a mockery of the government's proposal. However this is not to say that this is a definite description as proposed by the above statement.

D *The Home Office statistics are not a true representation of the total number of overseas workers.*

Answer: Can't tell

The statistics from the Home Office and the Department of Work and Pensions are of an inconclusive nature. However we are not given information which suggests that either statistic is a true representation of the total number of overseas workers.

Question 7

> *As she walked through the dark woods, she could feel the whisper of the wind blow across her face. The radiance of the sun peeked through the branches of the trees. The oak tree stood strong, facing the lake of swans. Towards the west stood an aged cottage house, amongst the perimeter of the building a pathway could be seen which led deeper into the darkness. Vanessa felt at peace, with the company of Mother Nature surrounding her. She walked towards the house and noted that towards her east stood a soaring fir tree. As she reached the doorstep of the house, she could see at the rear of the house the surface of Mount Sisilia. The ranges were intertwined but the two peaks could be briefly seen, which emphasised their individuality.*

A *The fir tree is on the left-hand side of the house.*

Answer: False

The fir tree is actually situated towards the 'east' of the house or the right-hand side rather than the left-hand side of the house.

B *Mount Sisilia consists of two mountain ranges.*

Answer: True

It is stated in the passage that the ranges were intertwined but the two peaks could be briefly seen, which suggests that there are two ranges which are closely merged together.

C   Opposite the lake is an oak tree.

Answer: True

It is stated in the passage 'The oak tree stood strong, facing the lake of swans'. Therefore 'facing' is used to describe the oak tree being positioned on the opposite side or facing the lake.

D   The character in the passage is not afraid of the woods.

Answer: Can't tell

In the passage it is stated that the character felt at peace with the company of Mother Nature; however we are not given information which suggests that she is or is not afraid, and therefore we are unable to conclude the above statement.

Question 8

> *The type and level of dyslexia varies from person to person. Approximately 60% of people with dyslexia suffer from phonological difficulties, and therefore have difficulty organising words from sounds, and the way they are written. This has often resulted in problems with reading, writing and spelling. One common feature is that people who have dyslexia often spell out words the way they sound, therefore making grammatical errors such as missing out silent letters and not following spelling rules.*
>
> *Dyslexia is usually noted in childhood, where children may confuse directional words and actions such as up and down, left or right, and in or out. During childhood they may also have difficulty with sequencing such as learning and memorising rhymes and number sequences.*
>
> *Dyslexia also continues throughout adulthood, and still affects sequencing and directional problems such as reading maps, difficulty with writing and reading tasks and dialling numbers on a telephone. Therefore, due to these difficulties with reading and spelling, individuals may find dictionaries and spell checkers difficult to understand.*

A   People with dyslexia may spell the word 'ghost' as 'gost, and miss out the letter 'H'.

Answer: True

Although this specific example is not given in the passage, it stated in the passage that people who have dyslexia may often 'spell out words the way they sound, therefore making grammatical errors such as missing out silent letters and not following spelling rules'. From this quote we are able to conclude the above statement as true, as there is a grammatical error from missing out the letter 'H'.

B   *Dyslexic children may have difficulty putting their shoes on correctly.*

Answer: True

As above the example is not given in the passage; however it is stated in the passage that a dyslexic child may find directional words and actions confusing, such as being able to tell their left from right. Therefore keeping this justification in mind, a dyslexic child may not be able to tell their left shoe from their right.

C   *Maps cannot help individuals who suffer from dyslexia.*

Answer: False

It is stated in the passage that people who have dyslexia can be affected by sequencing and directional problems such as reading maps; however this does *not* say that maps will not help them, therefore the answer is false.

D   *An individual who has dyslexia may find it difficult to write an essay.*

Answer: True

The above example is not illustrated in the passage, although it is stated in the passage that individuals may have difficulties with spelling and reading tasks. From this, we are able to use the example of writing an essay to illustrate such difficulties.

Question 9

> *Younger people were more likely to take days off due to sickness than older employees. This was the case for both gender groups. Amongst 16–25 year old men 2.6% were more likely to take days off due to sickness. Of women from the same age category; 3.5% were more likely to take days off due to sickness.*
>
> *Women with no dependant children had the same sickness absence as women who had dependant children. Women whose children were aged between 5–10 years were more likely to take sickness absence than men (3.6%).*
>
> *The employees most likely to be sick worked in professional and technical occupations at an absence rate of 3.2%. This was followed by a rate of 2.8% in the elementary occupations, such as hospital porters, window cleaners and traffic wardens. In comparison the rate for women was 4.2%.*

A **Women are more likely to take days off due to sickness than men.**

Answer: Can't tell

We are given many comparisons between the absenteeism levels between men and women, and at first it seems women seem to take more days off. In the second paragraph we are provided with information on sickness absenteeism of women with and without dependant children; although we are not given information about men who fit into the same category. Therefore there is insufficient information to conclude the above statement.

B **Employees of educational age are more likely to have sickness absences than older employees.**

Answer: Can't tell

Although we may know that young people aged 16–25 may be in education, we are not provided with this evidence in the passage and for this reason we are unable to conclude the above statement.

C **Professionals in stressful jobs, such as lawyers, are more likely to take days off.**

Answer: Can't tell

In the passage it is stated that people in professional jobs are more likely to take days off work. However, the above statement also adds the word 'stressful' and we are not provided with information which suggests that such jobs are stressful; therefore the answer is 'can't tell'.

D   *Young people take more sickness absence than older people.*

Answer: False

The above statement implies that young people will definitely take more sickness absence than older people; in contrast it is stated in the passage that young people are *more likely* to take sickness absence, therefore it is a possibility, rather than definite, that they will take more days off due to sickness.

Question 10

> *To be an effective leader, you need to have a vision and to know how you are going to bring people together to understand it. Charisma plays a vital role in leadership; charismatic leaders are admired by others and are concerned with others around them. A good leader also needs to understand when and when not to take risks, and how to portray success. Good leaders will usually pass down the glory to their teams, so that the teams feel satisfied with their winnings. When unforeseen circumstances come about, good leaders will also need to have the ability to claim a level of responsibility over strategies and related items which do not flow according to plan. True leaders are eager to offer power to get things done rather than hoarding power.*

A   *Good leaders should create a collective sense of achievement.*

Answer: True

The above statement is true as it is stated in the passage that 'Good leaders will usually pass down the glory to their teams, so that the teams feel satisfied with their winnings', which means that achievement or winnings should be collective or shared by all.

B   Good leaders should hand over complete power.

Answer: Can't tell

It is stated in the passage that 'true leaders are eager to offer power', but whether or not this means complete power is unknown and for this reason we are unable to conclude the above statement.

C   Charismatic leaders make better leaders.

Answer: Can't tell

From the passage we are given information that charisma plays a vital role in leadership, but whether or not this makes better leaders is not illustrated in the passage and for this reason we are unable to conclude the statement.

D   Good leaders will need to claim responsibility over events that do not go according to plan.

Answer: False

The statement suggests that good leaders will always need to claim responsibility over events that do not go according to plan; however in contrast to this it is stated in the passage that good leaders will need to _claim a level_, or a certain degree of responsibility. Therefore based on this information, the above statement is false.

Question 11

The Smoke-free law aims to improve health in many ways as it reduces the risk of individuals suffering from the effects of passive smoking. There are over 4,000 chemicals in second-hand smoke. These are in forms of particles and gases, which often have poisonous properties that are known to cause cancer and heart problems. Within 30 minutes of exposure to second-hand smoke, blood flow to the heart is restricted. The Smoke-free law aims to reduce such harmful effects of second-hand smoke.

The 'Smoke free law', passed by Parliament in 2006, makes virtually all enclosed public places and workplaces smoke-free. The law recognises individual rights to be protected from the harmful effects of smoke, and also aims to encourage smokers to quit. It has been suggested that reducing the exposure of cigarette smoke not only improves one's health, but also improves life expectancy.

> *There are limited exemptions from the smoke-free law. These regulations include bedrooms, hotels, care homes, prisons and various other 'live-in' premises. In the majority of cases, exemptions do not apply to the whole premises, but to certain 'designated rooms'.*

A   The smoke-free law will make people live longer.

Answer: Can't tell

We are given the aims and objectives of the smoke-free law; however there is no information which suggests that individuals will actually live longer for definite. Therefore we 'can't tell' whether people will live longer or not.

B   Night staff working in a residential home are allowed to smoke in their own bedrooms.

Answer: True

It is stated in the passage that exemptions only apply to certain designated rooms such as bedrooms and care homes.

C   There are 4,000 chemicals in second-hand smoke.

Answer: False

It is stated in the passage that there are **over** 4,000 chemicals in second-hand smoke, therefore there are **more** than 4,000 chemicals which contradicts the statement and makes it false.

D   Public places and workplaces will abide by the Smoke-free law.

Answer: Can't tell

The aim of this law is make 'enclosed public places and work places smoke-free', but whether or not these places will abide by the law is unknown as it is not stated in the passage. Therefore there is insufficient information to confirm the above statement.

Quantitative Reasoning Answers and Justifications

A = 5.2	B = 3.6	C = 7	D = 8	E = 0.01

Question 1   Answer A

Step 1 $D^3 \times C^2 = x^2$

Substitute the letters for numbers

$8^3 \times 7^2 = x^2$

Step 2   Work out the brackets

$x^2 = 512 \times 49$

$x^2 = 25088$

$x = \sqrt{25088}$

$x = 158.4$ **(to one decimal place)**

Question 2   Answer E

Step 1   Substitute the letters for numbers

$(A^3 - 3) \times 2.2 = x$

$(5.2^3 - 3) \times 2.2 = x$

Step 2   Simplify the formula

$(140.608 - 3) \times 2.2 = x$

$x = 302.7376$

The question for the value of x^2, not x

$x^2 = 302.7376^2$

$= 91650.05445$

$x^2 = 91650.1$ **(to one decimal place).**

Question 3   Answer E

Step 1   Substitute the letters for numbers

$(B \times C^2) \div 3 = x^2$

Step 2   First we need to work out the bracket

$(3.6 \times 49) \div 3 = x^2$

$176.4 \div 3 = x^2$

$x^2 = 58.8$

$x = 7.67$ (to two decimal places).

Question 4   Answer B

Step 1   Substitute the letters for numbers

$(D^2 - 6) + (14 \times B)$

$(8^2 - 6) + (14 \times 3.6) = x$

Step 2   Simplify the formula

$(64 - 6) + (50.4) = x$

$x = 58 + 50.4$

$x = 108.4$

The question asks us to find the value of x^3

$x^3 = 108.3^3$

$x^3 = 1273760.704$

$x^3 = 1273760.7$ (to one decimal place)

Question 5   Answer C

Step 1   Calculate the total ingredients required per person

Therefore 750 grams of flour ÷ 8 (people) = 93.75 grams per person.

Step 2   Multiply the amount per person by total number of servings.

93.75 grams of flour × 100 people = **9375 grams of flour for 100 people.**

Question 6   Answer A

Step 1   Calculate the amount of sugar required per person.

212.4 grams of sugar ÷ 8 (people) = 26.55 grams per person

Step 2   Multiply amount per person by total number of servings.

26.55 × 7 = 185.85 grams of sugar for 7 people.

= 185.85/1000

= **0.186 kilograms of sugar (to three decimal places)**

Question 7   Answer D

Step 1   Calculate the amount of ingredients required per person.

We already have the calculation of the amount of sugar per person (See above)

Step 2   Find 20% of the amount per person. To do this we divide the given percentage by 100 and then multiply the sum by the amount of sugar per person.

(20 ÷ 100) × 26.55 = 5.31

We then subtract this from the original amount.

26.55 − 5.31

= **21.24 grams of sugar per person.**

Question 8   Answer B

Step 1   In order to find out how many people the recipe will serve, we need to first calculate how much flour is required per person, which is 93.75 grams. (This has been previously calculated in Question 5).

We then divide the total amount of flour by the amount of flour per person

$1500 \div 93.75 = $ **16 people.**

Question 9   Answer C

The question requires you to find an average or the 'mean' of a game player's scores.

We calculate this by adding all the scores together and dividing the total number of games.

$(20 + 30 + 60 + 10 + 20 + 60 + 60 + 70 + 20 + 10) \div 10 = $ **36 (average or mean score).**

Question 10   Answer B

Step 1   Arrange all the numbers in an ascending order and find the middle value(s).

10, 10, 20, 20, **20, 30,** 60, 60, 60, 70

The median value lies between the two scores

$(20 + 30) \div 2 = $ **25 (median score).**

Question 11   Answer A

To work out the range of the scores, we need to subtract the lowest score from the highest score.

$70 - 10 = $ **60**

Question 12   Answer D

Step 1   We first need to find the mean score which is 36. This has been previously calculated in Question 9.

Step 2   We then need to calculate 12.3% of 36.

$(12.3 \div 100) \times 36 = 4.428$

Step 3   We then add the above total to the original mean score

$36 + 4.428 = 40.428$

$= \mathbf{40.43}$ (to two decimal places).

Question 13   Answer C

The question requires us to calculate how many green doors have a height of ≥ 600cm

$\geq$ This symbol simply means greater than or equal to.

There are 12 doors which have a height of 600 – 699 cm and 100 green doors which have a height of 700 – 799 cm. We then add the 2 values together to find the total number of green doors which have a height of $\geq$ 600 cm.

There are a total of 122 green doors which have a height of $\geq$ 600 cm.

Question 14   Answer C

Step 1   Calculate the number of blue doors which have a height of ≤ 499 cm and the number of yellow doors which have a height of ≤ 399 cm .

There are 56 blue doors with a height of $\geq$ 200 – 299 cm

There are 24 blue doors with a height of $\geq$ 300 – 399 cm

There are 42 blue doors with a height of $\geq$ 400 – 499 cm

In total there are 122 blue doors with a height of $\leq$ 499 cm

There are 12 yellow doors with a height of $\geq$ 200 – 299 cm

There are 22 yellow doors with a height of ≥ 300 – 399 cm

In total there are 34 yellow doors with a height ≤ 499 cm

The ratio of blue doors which have a height of ≤ 499 cm to the number of yellow doors which have a height of ≤ 399 cm is 122:34.

This value can be simplified by dividing by 2 to give the ratio

61:17

Question 15   Answer D

Step 1 Find the total number of yellow doors and the total number of doors altogether.

206 out of 2273 doors are yellow.

Step 2 We then calculate this as a percentage:

(206 ÷ 2273) × 100

= 9.06% of doors are yellow (to two decimal places).

Question 16   Answer A

Step First we need to calculate the number of green doors which have a height ≥ 600 cm.

There are 12/833 green doors which have a height of ≥ 600 – 699 cm.

And 110/833 green doors which have a height of ≥ 700 – 799 cm

So a total of 122 out of 833 green doors have a height ≥ 600 cm

Step 2 We then calculate this as a percentage (112 ÷ 833) × 100

= 14.65% (to two decimal places).

Question 17   Answer E

We know that 33% of 240 members of staff belong to the administration sector. We need to find the number of staff 33% of 240 represents:

(33 ÷ 100) × 240 (total number of staff) = 79.2 or **79 as a whole number.**

(It is better to use common sense when answering such questions as people can only be conveyed sensibly as whole numbers.)

Question 18   Answer B

Step 1   We first need to calculate how many members of staff there are in the banking sector.

(19 ÷100) × 240 = 45.6

Step 2   We then increase the number of staff in banking by 20%. This requires the following calculation:

(20 ÷ 100) × 46 = 9.2

Step 3   We then add 9.2 (the extra 20%) to the original number of staff in the banking sector:

9.2 + 45.6 = 54.8

= 55 (to the nearest whole number).

Question 19   Answer D

Step 1   We need to first calculate 21% of 240 to calculate the number of staff in the customer service sector:

(21 ÷ 100) × 240 = 50.4

Step 2   We then find 35% of these 50 members:

(35 ÷ 100) × 50.4 = 17.64

Step 3   We then add the above total to the original number of staff in customer service to find the new number of staff:

50.4 + 17.64 = 68.04 total number of staff in the customer service sector.

Step 4   We now need to convert the above total into a percentage. We need to add the extra number of staff members to the total number of staff employed. As noted in the calculations above there are 17.64 new members of staff to be added to the grand total of 240, making a new total of 257.64 staff.

Step 5   68.04 out of 257.64 members of staff are in the customer services department. As a percentage this is $(68.04 \div 257.64) \times 100 = 26.41\%$ **(to two decimal places).**

Question 20   Answer B

Step 1   Calculate the total numbers of staff there are in both banking and insurance (See Question 17).

In Insurance there are $(27 \div 100) \times 240 = 65$ members of staff

In Banking there are $(19 \div 100) \times 240 = 46$ members of staff

Step 2   Find the difference between the two totals: $65 - 46 = $ **19 more members in insurance than banking.**

A = −1	B = −3	C = 4.2	D = 5	E = 25.3	F = 3.9

Question 21   Answer E

$A + B^2 = x$

$-1 + (-3)^2 = x$

$-1 + 9 = x$

$x = 8$

$x^2 = 8^2$

$x^2 = 64$

Question 22   Answer A

$(C + B) \div F = x$

$(4.2 + -3) \div 3.9 = x$

$1.2 \div 3.9 = x$

$x = 0.307692307$

$x = 0.308$ (to three decimal places).

Question 23   Answer D

$E^2 + B^3 = \sqrt{x}$

$25.3^2 + (-3)^3 = \sqrt{x}$

$640.09 + -27 = \sqrt{x}$

$\sqrt{x} = 613.09$

$x = 375879.3$ (to one decimal place)

Question 24   Answer B

$D + C^2 \div F = x^2$

$5 + 4.2^2 \div 3.9 = x^2$

$x^2 = (5 + 17.64) \div 3.9$

$x^2 = 5.805128205$

$x = \sqrt{5.805128205}$

$x = 2.41$ (to two decimal places).

Question 25   Answer D

We first need to find the number of days lost as holiday and those that were lost due to sickness, and then find the difference between the two.

Holidays – 60

Sick Leave – 45

60 – 45 = **15 more holidays were taken.**

Question 26   Answer E

Step 1   First, we need to find the number of days lost due to maternity and paternity leave:

Maternity leave = 75, Paternity leave = 45

Therefore the ratio can be written as 75:45

Step 2   The above ratio can be reduced by a factor of 15.

$75 \div 15 = 5$

$45 \div 15 = 3$

This gives the ratio 5:3

Question 27   Answer B

Step 1   First we need to calculate the average number of days lost to sickness over the 3 months:

45 members of staff took sick leave over the 3 months

$= 45 \div 3$

$= 15$ days lost per month

Step 2   Month 4 sees a 33.3% increase in days lost to sickness, so we need to calculate 33.3% of 15:

$(33.3 \div 100) \times 15 = 4.995$

= 5 extra days lost in month four

Question 28   Answer C

Step 1   Find the loss per type of absence using the following formula:

(Number of staff × Loss per person)

Sick   45 × £47.00 = £2,115.00

Holidays   60 × £85.00 = £5,100.00

Maternity   75 × £80.00 = £6,000.00

Paternity   45 × £60.00 = £2,700.00

Grand total over 3 months = £15,915.00

Step 2   Find the average cost per month by dividing the total by 3

(£15,915.00 ÷ 3) = **£5,305 per month**

Question 29   Answer C

$150.00 ÷ 1.59 = **£94.34** (to two decimal places).

Question 30   Answer E

Step 1   We simply need to calculate the difference in dollars and express this as a percentage of the original value:

The difference between number of dollars you get

= 1.805 – 1.59

= 0.215 more dollars to the pound

Step 2   To express this as a percentage:

(0.215 ÷ 1.59) × 100

= **13.5% more dollars to the pound (to one decimal place)**

Question 31   Answer B

$120.00 ÷ £89.00 = **1.36** (to two decimal places).

Question 32   Answer A

£1 will give you 0.6 BGL, so £100.61 will give you

£100.61 × 0.6 = **60.37 BGL** (to two decimal places).

Question 33   Answer E

We use the method of reduction to find 27/108 in its simplest form.

The top number of a fraction is called a numerator; the bottom number is called a denominator.

Step 1   Divide both the numerator and denominator by the same number, until the numerator and denominator are as small as possible.

27/108 – If we divide this fraction by 3 we are left with 9/36. This fraction can still be reduced by 3, which then leaves us with 3/12; again we can still divide this number by 3, which now leaves the fraction in its smallest form: ¼

Question 34   Answer B

Step 1   We first need to convert the fractions so that the denominators are the same.

The easiest way to do this is to multiply each fraction by the denominator of the other fraction.

i.e 3/8 × 5 = 15/40

1/5 × 8 = 8/40

Step 2   As the denominators are the same we can simply add the two fractions and, if possible, reduce the answer to its lowest form

15/40 + 8/40

= **23/40**

Question 35   **Answer B**

11 ÷ 4 = 2 with a remainder of 3

= **2¾**

Question 36   **Answer A**

Multiply the whole number by the denominator: $3 \times 5 = 15$
Add the numerator to the product 15 + 2 = 17
Then write that down above the denominator as follows:
17/5

Question 37   **Answer C**

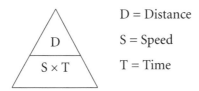

D = Distance

S = Speed

T = Time

Using   the above triangle, the question requires you to find the speed of a vehicle which travels 360 miles in four hours.

360 (distance) ÷ 4 (Time) = **90 miles per hour**

Question 38   **Answer A**

To work out the duration of a journey you need to divide the distance by speed.

Therefore 120 ÷ 60 = 2 hours or **120 minutes**

Question 39   Answer C

As above we need to calculate the time:

First journey = 150 ÷ 50 = 3 hours

Second journey = 160 ÷ 40 = 4 hours

This gives 7 hours in total or 420 minutes

There is also a resting time of 15 minutes which needs to be included as the question asks for the whole duration of the journey. 420 +15 = **435 minutes**

Question 40   Answer A

Step 1

We first calculate how long the first part of his journey was:

Distance = speed × time = 70 × 2 = 140 miles

Step 2

We then calculate how long the second part of his journey was:

Distance = speed × time = 30 × 1.5 = 45 miles

Then we simply add the two values together to give us the total distance travelled

= 140 + 45

=**185 miles**

Abstract Reasoning
Answers and Justifications

Question 1

Set A

There are 6 symmetrical shapes consisting of a rectangle, an oval, a smiley face, a heart, a cross and a 4 point star. All the shapes are drawn with a 'dashed' line. The rule in this set is that all the shapes must have at least *1 or more lines of symmetry.*

Set B

There are 6 non-symmetrical shapes, consisting of an arrow, a rectangle with a corner missing, a flag shape, a rounded speech bubble, an explosion symbol and a rectangle speech bubble. All the shapes are drawn with a 'dashed' line. The rule in this set is that all the shapes must have *no lines of symmetry.*

Test shape 1   Answer: Set A

The test shape belongs to Set A as there are 2 lines of symmetry. The shape could be symmetrical if 'folded' vertically or horizontally.

Test shape 2   Answer: Neither Set

The test shape consists of a 3D cube; it is not related to either set as both sets have a pattern of flat shapes.

Test shape 3   Answer: Set B

The test shape has no line of symmetry, and is therefore part of Set B. The test shape cannot be part of Set A, as there needs to be at least one line of symmetry.

Test shape 4   Answer: Set A

There is one line of symmetry which flows horizontally, therefore the shape flows logically from Set A.

Test shape 5   Answer: Neither Set

The outline of the shapes is 'dotted' rather than dashed; therefore this characteristic differs from the characteristics of both sets.

Question 2

Set A

In this set there is a combination of small hearts, stars, and circles. The rule in this set is where there are 3 stars, there should be 1 corresponding heart, and where there are 3 hearts there should be 1 corresponding star. The circles in this set are used as distracters.

Set B

As above in this set there is a combination of small hearts, stars, and circles. The rule in this set is where there are 4 circles, there should be 1 corresponding heart, and where there are 4 hearts there should be 1 corresponding circle. The stars in this set are used as distracters.

Test shape 1   Answer: Set A

This test shape belongs to Set A as there are 3 stars and 1 heart. It cannot be related to set B, as there needs to be 4 hearts to one circle, whereas in this test shape there is 1 heart to 4 circles.

Test shape 2   Answer: Set B

This test shape belongs to Set B, as there are 4 hearts to 1 circle. It cannot belong to Set A, as there needs to be 3 hearts instead of 4 hearts to 1 star.

Test shape 3   Answer: Set B

This test shape has 4 circles and 1 heart; therefore it has the corresponding patterns of Set B. It cannot be related to Set A, as there needs to be 3 hearts to 1 star to follow the rule, but this test shape has 1 heart to 4 stars.

Test shape 4   Answer: Neither Set

This test shape cannot be related to either set as there are only 2 of each shape.

Test shape 5   Answer: Set B

This test shape belongs to Set B, as there are 4 circles to 1 heart. It cannot belong to Set A, as there needs to be 1 heart to 3 stars.

Question 3

Set A

In this set there are various shapes made up of straight lines only. The rule in this set is that all the shapes should have 2 or more right angles. The remaining angles can be of any size.

Set B

There are various shapes made with straight and curved lines. The rule in this set is that each of the shapes must have only 1 right angle. The remaining angles in the shapes can be of any size.

Test shape 1   Answer: Neither

The shape has 2 right angles, therefore seems closer to Set A, however the shape cannot be part of Set A as it has a curved line- which is not a characteristic of Set A. The shape also does not belong to set B, as there are 2 right angles instead of 1.

Test shape 2   Answer: Neither

There are no angles within this test shape; hence it cannot belong to either Set.

Test shape 3   Answer: Group B

There is only 1 right angle in this test shape; therefore it follows the rule of Set B. It cannot be part of Set A, as there needs to be either 2 or more right angles in the test shape.

Test shape 4   Answer: Group A

There are 2 right angles in this test shape; therefore it follows the rule of Set A. It cannot be related to Set B, as the rule in this set allows for only 1 right angle per test shape.

Test shape 5   Answer: Neither

This test shape cannot go in either set, as there are no right angles.

Question 4

Set A

There are various shapes of various sizes, randomly assigned. Some are shaded in black, while others are in white. All the shapes are made with straight lines. There is only one rule to follow within this set. All the shapes must be made up of straight lines, regardless of size and colour. There should be no curved lines.

Set B

There are various shapes, of different sizes, all of which are randomly assigned. Again as in Set A, some are shaded in black whilst others are white. The only rule to follow in this set is that all the shapes must consist of only curved lines, regardless of shape, size and shading. There should be no straight lines.

Test shape 1   Answer: Neither Set

The shape cannot belong to either set, as it has a combination of straight and curved lines.

Test shape 2   Answer: Set B

All the shapes in this set are made up of curved lines only; therefore this test shape belongs to Set B.

Test shape 3   Answer: Set A

All the shapes in this set are made up of straight lines only; therefore this test shape belongs to Set A.

Test shape 4   Answer: Neither

The shape cannot belong to either set, as it has a combination of straight and curved lines.

Test shape 5   Answer: Set A

All the shapes in this set are made up of straight lines only; therefore this test shape belongs to Set A. There are no curved lines present, hence it cannot be part of Set B

Question 5

Set A

Within this set there are various shapes made with straight lines. The main rule in this set is that all the shapes must contain only 8 angles in total.

Set B

Within this set there are various shapes made with straight lines. The main rule in this set is that all the shapes must contain only 6 angles in total.

Test shape 1   Answer: Neither Set

The test shape does not belong to either set as it has a total of 7 angles.

Test shape 2   Answer: Set B

The test shape belongs to Set B, as there are a total of 6 angles.

Test shape 3   Answer: Set A

The test shape belongs to Set A, as there are a total of 8 angles.

Test shape 4   Answer: Set B

The test shape belongs to Set A, as there are a total of 6 angles.

Test shape 5   Answer: Set B

The test shape belongs to Set B, as there are a total of 6 angles.

Question 6

Set A

Within this set there are a number of different sized curved shapes. There is a repeating rule, in each box: there are 3 or 4 circular shapes, ranging from small, medium and large sizes. The *smallest* circular shape must always be inside the *largest* curved shape.

Set B

There are curved shapes, grouped in shapes of 3, 6 and 9. The shapes vary in either 2 or 3 different sizes in each of the boxes. The main rule is that the curved shapes must be in groups of 3, 6 *and* 9; in addition to this, the *smallest* curved shape must always be inside the *middle* sized curved shape.

Test shape 1   Answer: Set A

There are 3 different-sized curved shapes, ranging from small, medium and large. The smallest shape is inside the largest shape. This test shape cannot be part of Set B, as the smallest curved shape would have to be within the medium-sized shape.

Test shape 2   Answer: Neither

Again as above there are 3 curved shapes, ranging from small, medium and large. However the smallest shape is not within any of the circular shapes, therefore this test shape cannot be part of either set.

Test shape 3   Answer: Set B

There are 6 circular shapes, there is a 1 large oval shape, followed by 4 medium-sized circles, inside one of these medium sized circles there is a smaller circle within it. Therefore the shapes in this set are part of Set B, as they are in a group of 6, followed by the additional characteristic of the smallest shape being within the medium-sized shape. The set cannot belong to Set A, as the smallest shape would have to be within the largest shape.

Test shape 4   Answer: Set A

There are 4 different-sized curved shapes. The smallest curved shape is within the largest curved shape, making this pattern being similar to Set A. This test shape cannot be part of Set B, as the shapes are not grouped in 3, 6 or 9. As well as this, the smallest circle is not in the medium-sized curved shape; instead it is in the largest shape.

Test shape 5   Answer: Neither

Similarly to test shape 2, there are 3 curved shapes, ranging from small, medium and large. However the smallest shape is not within any of the circular shapes, therefore this test shape cannot be part of either set.

Question 7

Set A

There are various shapes made from straight lines. Some shapes are on their own, some are mixed with others. There are no curved shapes within this set. The rule in this set is that the shapes must be made from only *12 lines*.

Set B

Similar to the above set, there are various shapes made from straight lines. Some shapes are on their own, some are mixed with others. There are no curved shapes within this set. The rule in this set is that the shapes must only be made from 6 *lines.*

Test shape 1   Answer: Set A

The test shape belongs to Set A as the shape is made up of 12 lines.

Test shape 2   Answer: Neither Set

The test shape belongs to neither set as the shape is made up of 8 lines, instead of 12 or 6.

Test shape 3   Answer: Set A

The test shape belongs to Set A as the shape is made up of 12 lines.

Test shape 4   Answer: Set A

The test shape belongs to Set A as the shape is made up of 12 lines.

Test shape 5   Answer: Set B

The test shape belongs to Set B as the shape is made up of 6 lines.

Question 8

Set A

There are various shapes made up of both straight and curved lines. The shapes are either on their own or are paired with other shapes. Some of the shapes are in white, others are in black. The rule in this set is that the test shape must have at least one triangle, regardless of size.

Set B

There are various shapes made up of straight lines. The shapes are either on their own or are paired with other shapes. The shapes are all in white. The rule in this set is that *all* the test shapes must have at least one right angle regardless of size. There should be no triangular shapes within this set.

Test shape 1   Answer: Neither

The test shape looks close to set B, as there are 2 right angles. However, the second shape on the left-hand side is a heart and is therefore a curved shape. There are no curved shapes within this set. Additionally, this test shape cannot be part of Set A, as there are no triangles evident.

Test shape 2   Answer: Set A

The test shape is part of Set A, as there is a triangle which is attached to the rectangle on the right. This rectangle does have 4 right angles, there is an oval on the right-hand side, and this restricts the shape being part of Set B, as it is a curved shape.

Test shape 3   Answer: Set A

The test shape has a pentagon and a triangle; therefore it is part of Set A. It cannot be part of Set B, as there are no right angles within the shapes.

Test shape 4   Answer: Set B

The test shape consists of a square and a rectangle; both shapes have 4 right angles each, therefore the test shape is part of Set B. There are no triangles evident, and for this reason the test shape cannot belong to Set A.

Test shape 5   Answer: Set A

At first it seems the test shape can belong to both sets, as it contains both right angles and triangles. However at closer inspection, the rule of Set B is that *all* the shapes must have at least one right angle. However in this case, the 3 triangles do not contain any right angles, for this reason the most logical choice would be Set A.

Question 9

Set A

In this set, there are various-sized shapes made up of straight lines. There are no curved shapes in this set. Some of the shapes are coloured black, others are white. The shapes are also displayed either on their own or paired with other shapes. The main rule in this set is that the shape(s) in each box must have a total of *12 angles*, regardless of size.

Set B

As above, the set contains various shapes made up of straight lines of various sizes. There are no curved shapes in this set. Some of the shapes are coloured black, others are white. The shapes are also displayed either on their own or are paired with other shapes. The main rule in this set is that the shape(s) in each box must have a total of *6 angles*, regardless of size.

Test shape 1   Answer: Neither Set

The test shape has 8 angles; therefore it cannot belong to either group.

Test shape 2   Answer: Set B

The test shape has a total of 6 angles; for this reason it is part of Set B

Test shape 3   Answer: Set A

The test shape has a total of 12 angles, therefore it is part of Set A

Test shape 4   Answer: Set A

The test shape is part of Set A, as there are a total of 12 angles within the shape.

Test shape 5   Answer: Neither Set

The test shape contains a curved shape and therefore does not belong to either set, as both sets consist of shapes made from straight lines only.

Question 10

Set A

The set contains various sized squares, rectangles, and circular shapes. However each box in the set contains an arrow and a 24 point star which are of fixed sizes. Some of the shapes are coloured in black, others are in white. The rule in this set is that the 24 point star must always be placed close to the *corner* of the boxes, in the set. The arrow must always be situated towards the *left* hand side of each of the boxes and *point south*. The remaining shapes are randomly placed and are used as distracters.

Set B

The set contains the same shapes as Set A. There are various sized squares, rectangles, and circular shapes. However each box in the set contains an arrow and a 24 point star which are of fixed sizes. Some of the shapes are coloured in black, others are in white. The rule in this set is that the 24 point star must always be placed towards the *right*-hand side of the boxes. They should *never* be placed near the corners of the boxes. The arrow must always be situated either at the *top* or the *bottom* of the boxes, and must *point east*. The remaining shapes are randomly placed and are used as distracters.

Test shape 1   Answer: Set A

The test shape belongs to Set A, as the star is placed towards the bottom right-hand corner of the box, and the arrow is on the left-hand side pointing south. The test shape cannot belong to Set B, as the arrow is not at the top or the bottom of the box and it does not point east. The star is also situated at the corner of the box; therefore this restricts the test shape from being part of Set B.

Test Shape 2   Answer: Neither Set

The arrow points east, therefore in the first instance it may be possible to think that the test shape belongs to Set B. However at a closer analysis, the star is situated towards the left-hand corner of the box instead of being away from the corner towards the right-hand side of the box.
The test shape cannot belong to Set A, as the arrow points east instead of south.

Test shape 3   Answer: Set A

The arrow points south and is situated towards the left-hand side of the box. The star is also towards the right hand corner of the box. For these two reasons the test shape is part of Set A. The test shape cannot belong to Set B, as the star is situated in a corner, and the arrow does not point east.

Test shape 4   Answer: Set A

As above the arrow faces south and is situated towards the left-hand side of the box. The star is also towards the right hand corner of the box. For these two reasons the test shape is part of Set A. The test shape cannot belong to Set B, as the star is situated in a corner, and the arrow does not face east.

Test shape 5   Answer: Set B

The arrow faces east and is situated at the top of the box. The star is also towards the right and is not towards a corner. For these two reasons the test shape is part of Set B. The test shape cannot belong to Set A, as the star is not situated in a corner, and the arrow does not point south.

Question 11

Set A

The set contains various sized shapes made up of straight or curved lines. The shapes are either on their own or are randomly mixed with other shapes. There are no number patterns to follow. The only rule in this set is that in the test box there needs to be a *circle* present, regardless of size or number.

Set B

The set contains various sized shapes made up of straight or curved lines. The shapes are either on their own or are randomly mixed with other shapes. There are no number patterns to follow; the rules in this set are as follows in each box there is a large shape which is often manipulated with other shapes within it or surrounding it. The rule is to have the large shape replicated elsewhere in the box.

Test shape 1   Answer: Set B

The large heart shape is replicated into a smaller version on the outside of the shape. Therefore this test shape is part of Set B. It is not possible for this test shape to belong to Set A as there is an oval instead of a circle within the large heart shape.

Test shape 2   Answer: Set B

The large rectangle shape is replicated into a smaller version on the outside of the shape. Therefore this test shape is part of Set B. It is not possible for this test shape to belong to Set A as there are no circles present.

Test shape 3   Answer: Neither Set

The large shape is an oval and it is not replicated on the outside of the shape, hence it cannot be part of Set B. There are no circles present, and for this reason the test shape cannot belong to Set A.

Test shape 4   Answer: Set A

The test shape belongs to Set A, as there is a large circle, which has a distracter of a rectangle being inside it. The test shape cannot belong to Set B, as the large circle is not replicated on the outside of the shape.

Test shape 5   Answer: Set B

The large shape is replicated on the outside; therefore it belongs to Set B. The test shape also contains an oval; however it is important to remember not to get this confused with a circle. For this reason there are no circles in the test shape and hence it cannot be part of Set A.

Question 12

Set A

There are random symmetrical shapes, which are made up of both 'dashed' straight and curved lines. The main rule in this set is that each shape must be divided into 5.

Set B

There are random shapes which are made up of only 'dashed' straight lines. There are no curved shapes present. The rule in this set is that each shape(s) must have a total of 6 angles regardless of size.

Test shape 1   Answer: Set A

The test shape belongs to Set A, as the shape is symmetrical and is divided into 5 sections. The test shape cannot be part of Set B, as there are a total of 16 angles instead of 6 angles.

Test shape 2   Answer: Set B

The test shape has a total of 6 angles; therefore it belongs to Set B. It cannot belong to Set A, for 2 reasons: it is not divided into 5 sections and secondly, the second shape on the right is not symmetrical

Test shape 3   Answer: Set B

The test shape has a total of 6 angles and is therefore part of Set B. The test shape is not symmetrical and is not divided into 5; for this reason the test shape is not part of Set A.

Test shape 4   Answer: Neither Set

The test shape is not divided into 5 sections therefore it cannot be part of Set A. It also cannot belong to Set B, as there are a total of 8 angles instead of 6.

Test shape 5   Answer: Neither Set

As above, the test shape is not divided into 5 sections; therefore it cannot be part of Set A. It can also not belong to Set B, as there are a total of 8 angles instead of 6. As well as this, Set B does not contain any curved shapes.

Question 13

Set A

In this set there are small stars, hearts and triangles. There are two rules:

1 For every 4 stars there are 2 triangles.

2 For every 4 triangles there are 2 stars.

The hearts are used as distracters.

Set B

As above there are small stars, hearts and triangles. There are two rules:

1 For every 4 hearts there are 2 stars.

2 For every 4 stars there are 2 hearts.

The triangles are used as distracters.

Test shape 1   Answer: B

The test shape belongs to Set B, as there are 4 hearts to 2 stars. The test shape cannot belong to Set A, as there are 3 triangles instead of 4 triangles to 2 stars.

Test shape 2   Answer: B

The test shape belongs to Set B, as there are 4 stars to 2 hearts. The test shape cannot belong to Set A, as there are 3 triangles instead of 4 triangles to 2 stars.

Test shape 3   Answer: Neither Set

The test shape belongs to neither set, as there are only 2 triangles and 2 hearts but 6 stars, so this does not fit any of the combinations.

Test shape 4   Answer: Set A

The test shape belongs to Set A, as there are 4 stars to 2 triangles. The test shape cannot be part of Set B, as there are 7 hearts instead of 2 hearts to 4 star shapes.

Test shape 5   Answer: Set A

The test shape belongs to Set A, as there are 4 triangles to 2 stars. The test shape cannot be part of Set B, as there are 8 hearts instead of 2 hearts to 4 star shapes.

Decision Analysis
Answers and Justifications

Question 1   **Answer D**

L, (8, A), P, 3, ☹

The code combines the words: she, (attribute, sea), drop, past, listening

Option A   Does not make use of an 'attribute' or a characteristic of the 'sea' and is set in present tense.

Option B   Uses all the words in the code but does not make logical sense.

Option C   Ignores the word 'listening' and ignores 'attribute' of the sea.

Option D   **Is the correct answer. The statement is set in the past tense and uses all the codes. 'Drop' is substituted by the word 'falling', an attribute of the sea is water, therefore the word 'rain' is used to interpret the words in the brackets: (attribute, sea).**

Option E   Although an attribute of the sea could be waves, this statement is incorrect as it introduces the word 'music' and ignores 'drop'.

Question 2   **Answer B**

D, (8, B), (8, A), 3

The code combines the words: sun, (attribute, oxygen), (attribute, sea), past

Option A   This option uses most of the encoded words but it does not include an attribute of the sea.

Option B   **Is the correct answer as the sun and air (oxygen) is able to dry up water (rain, which is an attribute of sea). The statement is also set in the past tense.**

Option C   Ignores the words 'sun' and (attribute, sea) and is set in the present tense.

Option D	Ignores the words (attribute, sea) and introduces the word 'no'. Also set in present tense.
Option E	Introduces the word 'more'. Again, set in present tense.

Question 3   **Answer A**

4, (1, F), (1, E) H, D, 5

The code combines the words: future, (antonym, cold), (antonym, night), tomorrow, sun, increase

Option A   **Is the correct answer, as it uses all the words in the code and the enclosed rules within the brackets. The word 'very' is used to emphasise the heat (increase, heat), the antonym or opposite of cold is hot and the opposite of day is night.**

Option B	Ignores the word 'increased'.
Option C	There is a confusion of grammar; the statement uses both the present and future tenses.
Option D	Ignores the word 'sun'.
Option E	Ignores the word 'tomorrow'.

Question 4   **Answer B**

L, M, O, 5 (A, 8), 2

The code combines the words: she, run, building, increase, (sea, attribute), present

Option A	Introduces the word 'under', ignores 'increase' and is set in the past tense.
Option B	**Is the correct answer as it uses all the words within the code. The words 'sea' and 'attribute' are combined to give the word 'rain' and 'increased' is used to emphasise 'heavy rain'.**
Option C	Does not use the words 'increase' and (sea, attribute).
Option D	Introduces the word 'falling'.

Option E	This option is set in the future tense rather than the present tense, additionally the word 'falls' is introduced.

Question 5   Answer A

4, (A, 8), Q, (5, K), 9 (J, 7)

The code combines the words: future, (sea, attribute), jungle, (increase, hazard), conditional, (creature, plural)

Option A	**Is the correct answer, as it uses all the codes and the rules within the brackets. An attribute of the sea is 'flood' which is emphasised by 'increased hazard' or danger. The statement is also set in the future conditional tense.**
Option B	Is incorrect as it is set in the past tense rather than the future tense.
Option C	As above, this statement is set in the past tense and does not use attribute of the sea.
Option D	Changes creature and plural to inhabitants and is not in future conditional tense.
Option E	Set in the present tense rather than the future tense and ignores attribute of the sea.

Question 6   Answer B

(A, 8), (7, C, O), 2

The code combines the words: (sea, attribute), (plural, person, building), present

Option A	Does not combine the words (plural, person, building) and is set in the past tense.
Option B	**Although it introduces 'across' is the best match because it is set in the present tense and uses the words within the brackets. An attribute of the sea is lake, and the words (plural, person, building), are combined to give a public place or as interpreted in the statement 'church'.**
Option C	Does not combine the words (plural, person, building) and is set in the past tense.

Option D | Set in the past tense rather than the present tense.
Option E | As above this option is set in the past tense.

Question 7   **Answer E**

K, (7, C, O), (8, B), 3, R

The code combines the words: hazard, (plural, person, building), (attribute, oxygen), past, escape

Option A | Ignores all the words within the brackets.

Option B | Ignores combining the words (plural, person, building).

Option C | Uses all the words but is set in the present tense rather than the past tense.

Option D | Introduces the word 'avoided'.

Option E | **Is the correct answer, the combined words: (plural, person) building give the word 'office', and an attribute or characteristic of oxygen is 'gas'. The work 'leak' substitutes the word 'escape'.**

Question 8   **Answers A & C**

Ϋ, 9, (7, C), 3, (1, E), ☐

The code combines the words: brawling, conditional, (plural, person), past, (antonym, night), seeing

Option A | Uses all the words but introduces 'carried on'.

Option B | Introduces the word 'light'.

Option C | **Is the correct answer, as it combines the words (plural, person) as soldiers and are based on the condition that the soldiers would have only been able to fight had it been in the day (antonym, night).**

Option D | 'Seeing' is ignored, the statement is not based on a condition and adds in night in addition to day.

Option E | Ignores the word 'brawling' and adds in night in addition to day.

Question 9   **Answer C**

☹, (J, 7), (1, 11, N), L, 3

The code combines the words: listening, (creature, plural), (antonym, positive, emotion), she, past

Option A   Ignores the word 'listening'. Also it introduces 'saw' and 'come towards her'.

Option B   Ignores the word 'listening'.

Option C   **Is the right answer as the 'plural creature' is interpreted as 'animals', listening is substituted for 'heard' and (antonym, positive) emotion is interpreted as a negative emotion or as depicted in the statement ' frightened'.**

Option D   Does not make sense and ignores the word 'listening'.

Option E   Is set in the future tense rather than the past tense. As well as this the words 'coming towards her' are introduced.

Question 10   **Answer E**

S, (1, 5), 9 (1, ✎), (7, C), 2

The code combines the words: triumph, (antonym, increase), conditional, (antonym, trusting), (plural, person), present

Option A   Ignores the words (antonym, increase) and is set in the future and not on a conditional term.

Option B   Ignores the opposite of the words increase and trusting.

Option C   The statement is not set on a conditional term.

Option D   As above the statement is not set on a conditional term.

Option E   **Although it introduces the word 'we' is the most accurate interpretation as the sentence is based on the 'condition' if we are to doubt (antonym, trusting), each other (plural, person) then we are less likely (antonym, increase) to succeed (triumph).**

Question 11   **Answer D**

9, H, 5, (1, F), (7, C), A, 2, (5,   )

The code combines the words: conditional, tomorrow, increase (antonym, cold), (plural, person), sea, present, (increase, drinking)

Option A   Ignores the word 'increase' with hot and is set in future tense.

Option B   Ignores the words 'increase', 'tomorrow' and is not set on conditional terms.

Option C   Ignores the word 'increase' with hot and is set in future tense.

Option D   **Is the most accurate interpretation as it is based on the condition that people (plural, person) will drink a lot of water (increased, drinking) and (sea) if it is hot (antonym, cold) today. This statement is also set in the present tense.**

Option E   Ignores the word 'tomorrow'.

Question 12   **Answer A**

9, 4, S, (L, 1), ☦

The code combines the words: conditional, future, triumph, (she, antonym), smiling

Option A   **Is the correct answer. As it is based on the condition that he (she, antonym), will be happy (smiling) if he passes his exams (triumph). The statement is also based in the future conditional tense.**

Option B   Set in the past tense rather than the future tense.

Option C   Is not based on a conditional term.

Option D   Does not use the opposite of 'she'.

Option E   The statement is not based on conditional terms.

Question 13   Answer E

(C, 7, O), (C, 7), 3

The code combines the words: (person, plural, building), (person, plural), past

Option A	Is set in the future tense rather than the past tense.
Option B	Does not combine the words (person, plural) building.
Option C	As above the statement does not combine the words (person, plural, building).
Option D	Is set in the present tense rather than the past tense.
Option E	**Is the correct answer as the combined words in the bracket (person, plural, building) are interpreted as 'community centre', crowd of people replaces (person, plural) and finally the statement is set in the past tense.**

Question 14   Answer C

(7, C), R, Q, (K, J, 7)

The code combines the words: (plural, person), escape, jungle, (hazard, creature, plural).

Option A	Does not make the word 'person' plural.
Option B	Does not apply a word relating to a hazard towards the creatures/mammals.
Option C	**Is the most accurate answer. The words (hazard, creature) plural are replaced with 'dangerous animals', tribe replaces 'plural, person', escape is replaced with 'getaway' and 'rainforest' replaces jungle.**
Option D	Ignores the combined words (hazard, creature, plural).
Option E	Introduces the word 'quick'.

Question 15   Answer E

D, C (8, A), (N, 11) 5, (1, 11, N)

The code combines the words: sun, person, (attribute, sea), (emotion, positive) increase, (antonym, positive, emotion).

Option A   Does not include an attribute of a characteristic related to the sea. Also incorrectly substitutes people for person.

Option B   Ignores the combined words in the brackets which describe a negative emotion (antonym, positive, emotion).

Option C   Ignores the combined words which describe an increase of a positive emotion (emotion, positive) increase.

Option D   In the same way as Option A, this option also does not include an attribute of a characteristic related to the sea.

Option E   Is the correct answer as: I (person) feel very happy (an increase of a positive emotion) when it is sunny (sun), and sad (negative emotion) when it rains (characteristic of sea).

Question 16   Answers B & C

(1, 11,) N, C, (A, ⚌) ⚌

The code combines the words: (Antonym, positive) emotion, person, (sea, dining), dining

Option A   Does not apply the rules of finding the opposite meaning to a positive emotion.

Options B & C   These two are the correct interpretations as they use all the words within the codes and the rules within the brackets.

Option B is correct as, I (person) dislike (antonym, positive) emotion, the taste (dining) of fish (sea, dining).

Option C is also a correct interpretation as I (person) dislike (antonym, positive) emotion, the taste (dining) of sea food (sea, dining).

Option D	Is incorrect as it does not use the rules of finding the opposite meaning to a positive emotion.
Option E	Does not combine the words 'sea, dining' together.

Question 17   **Answer E**

(C, 7), (I, 7) 3, ℣

The code combines the words: (person, plural), (weapon, plural), past, brawling

Option A	Ignores the rules of combining (person, plural) and uses 'I' instead. In addition to this, this option also ignores the word 'weapon'.
Option B	As above the statement ignores the rules of combining (person, plural) and uses 'I' instead.
Option C	Is set in the future tense.
Option D	Is set in the future tense and ignores the words (weapon, plural).
Option E	**Is the most accurate interpretation, as soldiers replaces 'plural person', arms replaces 'weapons', conflict replaces 'brawling' and finally the statement is set in the past tense.**

Question 18   **Answer D**

2, (7, C), ♌, ♌

The code combines the words: present, (plural, person), trusting, conversing

Option A	Introduces 'never' and portrays the word 'trusting' in a negative way.
Option B	Ignores the combination of the words 'plural, person'.
Option C	As above the statement ignores the combination of the words 'plural, person'.

Option D	Although it introduces 'maintain' and 'important' is the best match because it combines the words 'plural, person' and is interpreted in the statement as 'staff'. The words 'communicate verbally' replaces 'conversing' and finally the statement is set in the present tense.
Option E	Introduces the word 'listen'.

Question 19   Answer B

5(8, A), (7, C, O), K, 4

The code combines the words: increase (attribute, sea), (plural, person, building), hazard, future

Option A	Is set in the past tense rather than the future tense and does not combine the words (plural, person, building).
Option B	**Is the most accurate answer as it substitutes the code increase (attribute, sea) for flood which is an increase in water. The word 'dangerous' replaces hazard and 'library' replaces the combined words in brackets (plural, person) building.**
Option C	Is set in the past tense and does not use an attribute or a characteristic of the sea.
Option D	Ignores the combination of the words (plural, person, building).
Option E	In a similar way to Option C, Option E also does not use an attribute or a characteristic of the sea.

Question 20   Answer E

C, (1, 11),   , 13, (7, C,   ), 5

The code combines the words: person (antonym, positive), drinking, frequently, (plural, person, drinking), increase

Option A	Uses drinking in a positive light e.g. 'I like' rather than in a negative perspective as suggested by the code (opposite, positive).
Option B	Is incorrect as it does not combine the words (plural, person, drinking) increase.
Option C	Does not include opposite of positive in relation to drinking.
Option D	Is incorrect as it does not combine the words (plural, person, drinking) increase, or include the opposite of positive.
Option E	**Is the best interpretation as it combines all the words and uses all the rules within the brackets. 'I (person) do not enjoy (opposite of positive) regularly drinking (drinking, frequently) or socialising with others (plural person drinking) increase'.**

Option 21   Answer A

C, 9, ✞, 4, ☺, ♌

The code combines the words: person, conditional, smiling, future, listening, conversing

Option A	**Is the correct answer as it is based on the condition that 'I (person) will be (future) happy (smiling) to speak (conversing) to you only if (conditional) you listen (listening) to what I have to say (conversing)'.**
Option B	The statement is not set on a conditional term.
Option C	Ignores the word 'smiling'
Option D	Introduces the word 'creature'.
Option E	Repeats the words 'person', 'conditional' and 'present'.

Option 22	**Answer D**
	(7, C), (7, J), P, 2, (1, F)
	The code combines the words: (plural, person), (plural, creature), drop, present, (antonym, cold)
Option A	Does not include a code to describe the word 'dropping'.
Option B	Does not include codes which describe the words 'heat' and 'dropping'.
Option C	Does not include the code to describe the word 'dropping' and does not use brackets to give specific meanings to pairs of codes such as (plural, creature).
Option D	**Is the most accurate interpretation as: 'people (plural, person), are dropping (drop) like flies (plural, creature) from the heat (antonym, cold)'.**
Option E	Does not include the code to describe 'people' and uses the code to describe 'person' (C) instead.

Option 23	**Answer A**
	✧, ✿
	The code combines the following words: smiling, cope
Option A	**Is the best interpretation as it portrays the sentence into its simplest form: 'grin (smiling) and bear (cope) it'.**
Option B	Introduces the code for the word 'creature'.
Option C	Unnecessarily repeats the code for 'cope' (✿)
Option D	Does not use a code to describe the word 'grin' and introduces the code for the word 'sea' (A).
Option E	Combines codes together unnecessarily.

Question 24   Answer B

(A, T), (1, 12), G, K, 2

The code combines the words: (sea, move), (antonym, weak), today, hazard, present

Option A	Includes brackets around pairs of codes, unnecessarily and incorrectly.
Option B	**Is the correct answer as it is set in the present tense and interprets the sentence in the following way: 'The tide (sea, move) is very strong (antonym, weak) today and is dangerous (hazard).**
Option C	Does not include a code to describe the sentence being set in the 'present' tense. The code for the word 'future' (4) is used instead.
Option D	Does not include a code to describe the word 'strong' instead uses the code for 'weak'.
Option E	Does not use brackets to give specific meanings to pairs of codes.

Question 25   Answer C

L, Ƴƀ, 3, B, M, O

The code combines the words: she, brawling, past, oxygen, run, building

Option A	Does not include a code which describes the word 'breath'.
Option B	Unnecessarily repeats the following codes: 'L' and '3'.
Option C	**Provides the best interpretation of the sentence: 'She was fighting (brawling) for breath (oxygen) as she ran (run) home (building)'. The sentence is also based in the 'past' tense.**
Option D	Does not include a code which describes the word 'fighting'.
Option E	Does not include a code which suggests the sentence is based in the 'past' tense. Instead the code for 'future' (4) is used .

Question 26   Answer E

(1, L), 3, ✟,   , 2

The code combines the words: (antonym, she), past, smiling, seeing, present

Option A   Does not include a code to describe the word 'he' and uses the code for 'she' (L) instead.

Option B   Does not include brackets to give specific meanings for 'he' (1, L).

Option C   Does not use a code to describe the word 'happy'.

Option D   Introduces a code for the word 'cold' (F).

Option E   Is correct as it provides the most accurate interpretation of the sentence. 'He (antonym, she) was happy (smiling) to see (seeing) his gift (present)'.

Chapter 9

Closing Thoughts

The aim of this guide has been to provide you with an insight into the UKCAT and give you the opportunity to practise the various questions you will come up against. Our hope is that, by following the principles and steps contained in this guide, you will confidently be able to complete your UKCAT with excellent results.

If you feel that you still require further practice and would like to experience the UKCAT in an online format, you can subscribe to our online revision lessons at www.apply2medicine.co.uk.

In addition to this guide, the Apply2Medicine website contains lots of free resources, including details of 'hot topics' in the medical and dental world, to help you prepare for your application to Medical or Dental School and subsequent interview.

We strongly recommend that you do seek more information from the Medical or Dental Schools to which you are applying, and also from the official UKCAT websites, to ensure that you are fully prepared for your UKCAT.

From all at Apply2Medicine we would like to wish you every success in securing your place at Medical or Dental School.

Good Luck!

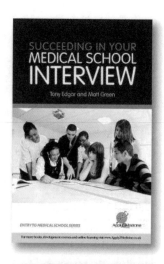

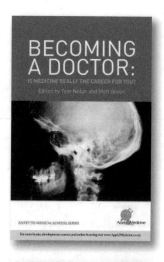

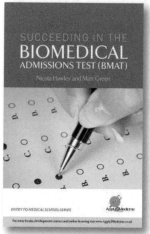

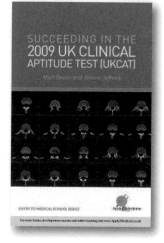

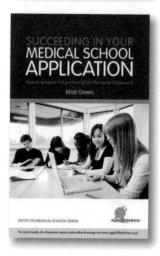

ENTRY TO MEDICAL SCHOOL SERIES

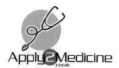

Apply2Medicine
.co.uk

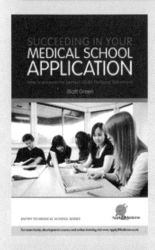
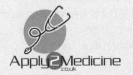

More titles in the Entry to Medical School Series

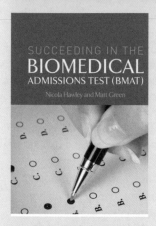

February 2009

200 pages

Paperback

978-1-906839-00-0

Succeeding in the Biomedical Admissions Test (BMAT) contains detailed guidance, practice questions and a complete mock test, to help applicants, parents and teachers alike to prepare for and successfully complete the BMAT. In this guide, Nicola Hawley and Matt Green:

- Describe the context of the BMAT within the application process

- Set out how to approach the three sections of the BMAT – namely the Aptitude and skills, Scientific Knowledge and Applications and the Written tasks

- Provide practice questions for each section to work through as part of the learning process

- Explore time management techniques to ensure optimal performance

- In addition provide a full mock exam for readers to complete under test conditions

This engaging, easy to use and comprehensive guide is essential reading for anyone serious about excelling in their BMAT examination and successfully securing their place at university.

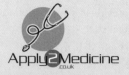

More titles in the Entry to Medical School Series

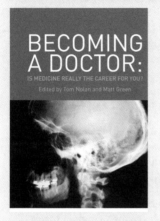

BECOMING A DOCTOR:
IS MEDICINE REALLY THE CAREER FOR YOU?
Edited by Tom Nolan and Matt Green

January 2009

152 pages

Paperback

978-0-9556746-6-2

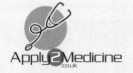

Deciding on whether or not to pursue a career in medicine is a decision that should not be taken lightly. Becoming a doctor can be highly rewarding but is not without its drawbacks. It is therefore important that you gain a clear insight into the world of medicine to ensure that it is the right path for you to follow.

This book has been written with the above in mind to provide a clear picture of what becoming a doctor really involves. In this comprehensive book Matt Green and Tom Nolan explore:

- What it really means to be a good doctor
- The steps that should be taken to confirm whether a career in medicine is really the one for you
- How to successfully apply to medical school including the various entrance exams (UKCAT, BMAT, GAMSAT), the UCAS personal statement and subsequent medical school interview
- Life as a student at medical school and how to excel
- The various career paths open to you as a doctor with invaluable insights provided by practising doctors.

This engaging, easy to use and comprehensive book is essential reading for anyone serious about becoming a doctor and determining whether it really is the right career for you!

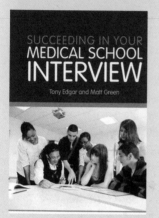
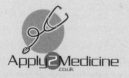